Radioactive Sample Counting: Principles and Practice (Second Edition)

IPEM report 85

IPEM–IOP Series in Physics and Engineering in Medicine and Biology

About the Series

The series in Physics and Engineering in Medicine and Biology will allow the Institute of Physics and Engineering in Medicine (IPEM) to progress its mission to 'advance physics and engineering applied to medicine and biology for the public good'.
It is focused on key areas including, but not limited to:

- clinical engineering
- diagnostic radiology
- informatics and computing
- magnetic resonance imaging
- nuclear medicine
- physiological measurement
- radiation protection
- radiotherapy
- rehabilitation engineering
- ultrasound and non-ionising radiation.

A number of IPEM–IOP titles are being published as part of the EUTEMPE Network Series for Medical Physics Experts.

A full list of titles published in this series can be found here: https://iopscience.iop.org/bookListInfo/physics-engineering-medicine-biology-series.

Radioactive Sample Counting: Principles and Practice (Second Edition)

IPEM report 85

Edited by
Sofia Michopoulou
University Hospital Southampton NHS Foundation Trust, Southampton, UK

With contributions from:
Andrew Fenwick
National Physical Laboratory, Teddington, UK

Fergus McKiddie
Nuclear Medicine Department, Aberdeen Royal Infirmary, Foresterhill, Aberdeen, UK

Peter O'Sullivan
North Cumbria Integrated Care NHS Foundation Trust, UK

Lucy Pike
King's College London, PET Centre, St Thomas' Hospital, London, UK

Anne-Marie Stapleton
Royal Surrey NHS Foundation Trust, Nuclear Medicine Department, St Luke's Cancer Centre, Royal Surrey County Hospital, Guildford, Surrey, UK

IOP Publishing, Bristol, UK

ISBN 978-0-7503-3895-0 (ebook)
ISBN 978-0-7503-3893-6 (print)
ISBN 978-0-7503-3896-7 (myPrint)
ISBN 978-0-7503-3894-3 (mobi)

DOI 10.1088/978-0-7503-3895-0

Version: 20220701

IOP ebooks

British Library Cataloguing-in-Publication Data: A catalogue record for this book is available from the British Library.

Published by IOP Publishing, wholly owned by The Institute of Physics, London

IOP Publishing, Temple Circus, Temple Way, Bristol, BS1 6HG, UK

US Office: IOP Publishing, Inc., 190 North Independence Mall West, Suite 601, Philadelphia, PA 19106, USA

Contents

Radioactive Sample Counters Working Group 2021

A Fenwick, F McKiddie, P O'Sullivan, L Pike, and A-M Stapleton

This is the second edition of *Radioactive Sample Counting—Principles and Practice*. Certain figures, tables, graphs, and passages of text included within this book have been reproduced from the first edition. The bibliographic details of the first edition are included below:

Radioactive Sample Counting—Principles and Practice

Edited by Ian Driver, © The Institute of Physics and Engineering in Medicine 2002

Report 85*: Radionuclide Special Interest Group* 2002

J Fleming, N Williams, J Skrypniuk, P Thorley, M Rose, I Driver, and B Murby

TGR33: Radionuclide Topic Group 1980

J H Todd (Chairman and Report Editor), M D Short, R G Bessent, L A Hawkins, K G Leach, D Ottewell, and D W Morgan.

Preface

This report originates from the TGR33 document produced by the Radionuclide Topic Group of the Hospital Physicists' Association (HPA) in 1980. In 2002, IPEM's Radionuclide Special Interest Group updated the document and produced Report 85.

In 2021, IPEM's Radioactive Sample Counters Working Group updated the report further, producing a handbook for joint publication by IOP and IPEM. The latest version has been restructured with separate chapters for the different types of counting equipment and covers instrumentation, applications, and quality assurance.

Many of the aims of this handbook remain the same as those of Report 85, specifically:

1. to provide a concise description of the basic design of radioactivity counters
2. to describe the facilities available for data analysis and presentation
3. to identify parameters which are important during daily use
4. to suggest factors which should be considered when purchasing a counter

The original material has been restructured to focus on the different types of equipment in use and extended to include detailed sections on:

1. quality control charts
2. quality assurance of gamma counters and scintillation detection systems
3. instrumentation and quality assurance of gamma probes
4. instrumentation and quality assurance of blood sampling systems
5. practical examples of sample counting for clinical and research applications

This handbook should be a valuable reference source for staff in a variety of professions who require a fundamental understanding of the processes involved in the absorption and detection of ionising radiation using sample counters. Indeed, the chapters covering the detection of radiation and nucleonic equipment are equally applicable to understanding the principles of photon detection in gamma cameras. Additionally, this handbook can be used as a guide for equipment procurement and quality assurance. Finally, it should be a helpful source of information when designing counting protocols and planning analysis of results.

List of abbreviations

ADC	Analogue to digital converter
ARSAC	Administration of Radioactive Substances Authorisation Committee
BNMS	British Nuclear Medicine Society
BSA	Body surface area
CsI	Caesium iodide
CsSb	Caesium antimony
CdTe	Cadmium telluride
CZT	Cadmium zinc telluride
CE	European conformity
CEIP	Compton edge inflexion point
CPM	Counts per minute
CPS	Counts per second
CT	Computed tomography
DRL	Diagnostic reference level
DSPs	Digital signal processors
DPM	Disintegrations per minute
DC	Direct current
EC	European Commission
EPR	Environmental permitting regulations
ESCR	External standard channels ratio
FDG	Fluorodeoxyglucose
FPGAs	Field-programmable gate arrays
FWHM	Full width at half maximum
FWTM	Full width at one-tenth maximum
GaP	Gallium phosphide
GFR	Glomerular filtration rate
GMP	Good manufacturing practice
HV	High voltage
IRR	Ionising Radiations Regulations
IRMER	Ionising Radiation Medical Exposure Regulations
LAN	Local area network
LLD	Lower-level discriminator
LSC	Liquid scintillation counting
MCA	Multichannel analyser
MDA	Minimum detectable activity
MDR	Medical Devices Regulations
MPE	Medical physics expert
MR	Magnetic resonance
MSB	Most significant bit
NaI	Sodium iodide
NEMA	National Electrical Manufacturers Association
NTP	Network time protocol
PET	Positron emission tomography
PMT	Photomultiplier tube
QA	Quality assurance
QC	Quality control
QE	Quantum efficiency

ROI	Region of interest
SCR	Sample channels ratio
SCA	Single channel analyser
SD	Standard deviation
SiPM	Silicon photomultiplier
SIS	Spectral index of sample
SPECT	Single-photon emission computed tomography
SQP(I)	Spectral quench parameter of the isotope
TAC	Time–activity curve
UPS	Uninterruptible power supply
ULD	Upper-level discriminator
UV	Ultraviolet
WEEE	Waste Electrical and Electronic Equipment

List of contributors

Andrew Fenwick
National Physical Laboratory, Teddington, UK

Fergus McKiddie
Nuclear Medicine Department, Aberdeen Royal Infirmary, Foresterhill, Aberdeen, UK

Sofia Michopoulou
University Hospital Southampton NHS Foundation Trust, Southampton, UK

Peter O'Sullivan
North Cumbria Integrated Care NHS Foundation Trust, UK

Lucy Pike
King's College London, PET Centre, St Thomas' Hospital, London, UK

Anne-Marie Stapleton
Royal Surrey NHS Foundation Trust, Nuclear Medicine Department, St Luke's Cancer Centre, Royal Surrey County Hospital, Guildford, Surrey, UK

Chapter 1

Physical principles of radiation detection in sample counters

Sofia Michopoulou

1.1 Introduction

There are currently many clinical applications, both routine and research, that involve assessing the radioactivity in samples of body fluids. These include radioimmunoassay, body volume measurements, and tracer kinetic studies of absorption and clearance.

Most sample counters detect radiation by scintillation spectrometry, in which gamma-ray, alpha-, or beta-particle energy is converted into light photons by a detector. The first use of this process was by Crookes and Regener (Birks 1964), who in 1908 detected alpha particle interactions in zinc sulphide by visual observation of the light emitted. The invention of the photomultiplier tube (PMT), which enabled the light energy to be converted into an electrical pulse, greatly enhanced the ability of scintillators to count particle interactions (Blau and Dreyfus 1945). At around the same time, new scintillators were discovered, including thallium-activated sodium iodide (NaI(Tl)) (Hofstadter 1949) and organic liquids (Kallmann 1950); these soon became established as valuable for counting gamma and beta samples, respectively (Anger 1951, Raben and Bloembergen 1951). Alternative scintillator materials include thallium-activated caesium iodide (CsI(Tl)), which is routinely used in gamma probe systems, as described in chapter 5.

More recently semiconductor detectors, such as cadmium telluride (CdTe) and cadmium zinc telluride (CZT), have been used in intraoperative gamma probes. Their compact size and excellent energy resolution (Zanzonico and Heller 2000) makes them suitable for intraoperative measurements of radioactivity to help pinpoint the locations of small regions of clinical interest (such as lymph nodes) *in vivo* and facilitate minimally invasive node resection. Automatic blood sampling systems that

doi:10.1088/978-0-7503-3895-0ch1

use a pump and online sample counters have become available, facilitating real-time assay of radioactivity in blood for tracer kinetic studies. These are mostly used with short-lived radionuclides for PET pharmacokinetic studies.

The counting of gamma or x-ray emitters is accomplished by external detection, as their photons readily pass through the sample material and the vial wall. Detectors made of solid materials with high atomic numbers are preferred, due to their high counting efficiency. They should ideally also be able to measure the energy loss of events to allow different emissions to be separately identified. Inorganic scintillators fit these requirements well, among which NaI(Tl) is the best suited for gamma sample counters. Semiconductor detectors have superior energy resolution when compared to inorganic scintillators, but generally have significantly lower counting efficiency.

The counting of beta emitters is more difficult, as the energy of the particles is efficiently absorbed in the sample material and the vial wall. Liquid scintillation counting is the principal method used for assaying beta-emitting samples, as the scintillants can be mixed with the sample. The beta particles are then detected in the scintillator before they lose any energy in intervening attenuating material, so providing a 4π solid-angle counting geometry. It is also possible to use liquid scintillators for alpha particle and gamma-ray detection. Liquid scintillation counting is described in chapter 6.

1.2 Light-emitting processes

Scintillators detect radiation by the process of luminescence, which is the emission of light from a material in which electronic excitations have occurred. These excitations may arise from the absorption of nuclear radiation, but can also be caused by such processes as light absorption, chemical reactions, thermal heating, and electrical discharge.

1.3 Sodium iodide detectors

The detector used in most modern gamma counters is a single crystal of NaI(Tl). This has been the detector of choice for gamma counting since its invention in the late 1940s (Hine 1967). Pure sodium iodide scintillates only at low temperatures; however, the incorporation of thallium impurity atoms at a concentration of about 0.2% produces crystal imperfections, known as luminescence centres, which can be excited by ionising radiation at room temperature (Birks 1964).

The selection of NaI(Tl) is based on several physical properties:

- A density of 3.67 g cm^{-3} and an effective atomic number of 50 make it an efficient absorber of low- and medium-energy gamma rays up to $\approx$300 keV.
- It provides a signal which is proportional to the energy lost in the crystal and can therefore be used for energy-selective counting.
- It has a relatively high yield of $\approx$40 photons per keV of absorbed energy at room temperature, giving an energy resolution which is adequate for most applications of sample counters.

- It has a decay time of 0.23 μs. This enables reasonably high count rates to be achieved without significant dead-time loss, although this is a limitation in some applications of the detector.
- It is transparent and therefore large detectors can be constructed without significantly reducing the amount of light detected.

However, it does have some disadvantages which have to be considered in the design and use of detectors. The crystals are quite fragile and may be fractured by mechanical pressure or by temperature change (see section 4.6.5). NaI(Tl) is also hygroscopic, and exposure to the atmosphere produces yellow discoloration which attenuates the light output. For these reasons the crystal is sealed in an aluminium case. Even a sealed crystal eventually undergoes yellowing and this ultimately limits the lifetime of a detector to around 10–15 years. The environment of the detectors also has to be carefully controlled, in particular to avoid rapid temperature change.

1.3.1 Primary interaction processes

Gamma rays passing through the crystal are initially attenuated by photoelectric, Compton, or pair-production interactions.

The photoelectric effect is an event in which the gamma ray transfers all its energy to an inner orbital electron of an atom, resulting in the ejection of a bound electron. The electron is slowed down in the sodium iodide crystal by collisions with other electrons and becomes part of the general electron population. Some of this kinetic energy is transformed into light, as described in more detail below.

Compton scattering occurs when a gamma ray interacts with an outer orbital electron, which is regarded as a free electron. The photon is scattered with reduced energy and its energy loss is transferred to the electron as kinetic energy.

Pair production is an event which occurs in the high electric field close to the nucleus of an atom. The gamma-ray energy is converted to mass and creates an electron–positron pair. This can only occur for gamma-ray photons with a minimum energy of 1.02 MeV, the energy equivalent of the rest mass of the electron–positron pair. Any energy in excess of 1.02 MeV is partitioned as kinetic energy between the two particles. Both the electron and positron are slowed down, rapidly losing their kinetic energy in collisions with absorber electrons. The positron then undergoes annihilation with one of the electrons. The mass of the two particles is converted into energy, producing two gamma photons, each with an energy of 511 keV which are emitted at approximately 180° to each other. In crystals of the typical size used in gamma counters, these annihilation photons have a reasonably high probability of escaping from the detector without interaction.

The relative importance of these absorption processes for various gamma-ray energies is shown figure 1.1, which is a plot of the respective absorption coefficients against gamma-ray energy for both NaI(Tl) and organic liquid scintillators (sections 1.3 and 1.4).

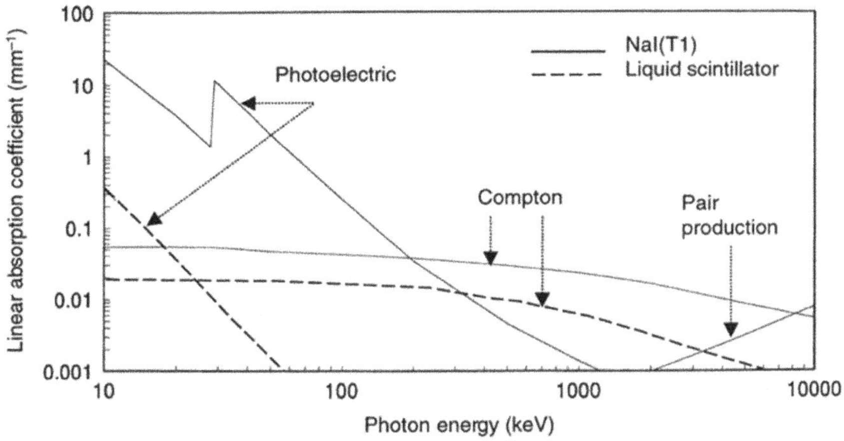

Figure 1.1. Energy dependence of the absorption processes for NaI(Tl) and organic liquid scintillator.

1.3.2 Secondary interaction processes

Each of the primary interaction processes produces an energetic secondary electron, which loses energy by exciting other electrons in the crystal from the ground state to the conduction band, creating electron–hole pairs. As these excited electrons return to the ground state, they give rise to photons in the wavelength range of 300–500 nm. This range is partly in the visible region of the electromagnetic spectrum and partly in the near-UV region. About 20–30 photons are produced per keV of energy loss. Most of the rest of the energy is dissipated as heat. The number of photons produced is proportional to the energy lost by the gamma ray in the crystal. The intensity of luminescence is temperature dependent, with an energy peak that increases in size with decreasing detector temperature. For NaI(Tl) the decay time of luminescence is 0.23 μs. The light photons are detected by a PMT which converts their energy to a pulse in an electrical circuit, the size of which is proportional to the light detected by the photocathode (section 2.2).

1.3.3 The pulse size spectrum

A spectrum of pulses is produced as a result of the different interaction processes undergone in the detector. The voltage values of the pulse heights are converted to energy losses in keV. A typical spectrum for ^{137}Cs obtained from a 50 mm × 50 mm NaI(Tl) crystal is shown in figure 1.2, which illustrates some of the common features listed below. For further information on the pulse size spectrum, see chapter 10 of Physics in Nuclear Medicine (Cherry *et al* 2012).

1. *Photopeak:* two main processes contribute to the photopeak:
   (a) *Photoelectric:* the total energy of a gamma ray is absorbed in the scintillator by the initial photoelectric event, followed by absorption within the scintillator of any resulting scattered electrons and x-rays, giving rise to a full-energy peak (photopeak).

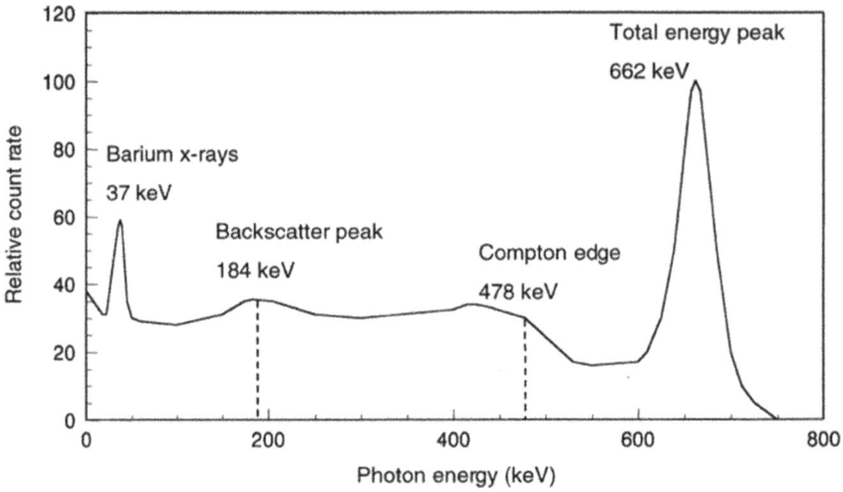

Figure 1.2. Gamma-ray spectrum of ^{137}Cs in a sodium iodide (Tl) detector.

(b) *Compton:* the total energy of a gamma ray is absorbed in the scintillator by a single or multiple Compton scattering events, followed by a photoelectric event. The probability of such absorption increases with crystal thickness.

2. *Compton plateau:* during Compton scatter events, when the scattered photon escapes the detector without further interaction, the energy deposited in the crystal is less than that of the photopeak and depends on the scatter angle. This process gives rise to the Compton continuum. The continuum includes a broad spectrum of pulse sizes, corresponding to the variable energy of the secondary electrons produced by the Compton scattering process. The upper limit of the secondary electron energy corresponds to a photon scattering angle of 180° and gives rise to a feature known as the Compton edge.
3. *Barium x-ray peak:* many gamma-emitting radionuclides have an alternative decay path by internal conversion which results in the emission of a characteristic x-ray from the daughter nucleus. In the case of ^{137}Cs, this is a barium x-ray at 37 keV.
4. *Backscatter peak:* this occurs when the gamma rays are backscattered into the scintillator after undergoing a Compton scattering event in the surrounding materials. The energy of the backscatter peak is approximately equal to the energy of a 180° Compton-scattered photon and approaches a maximum of 0.25 MeV as the energy of the incident gamma ray increases.

   Lead peak: Photoelectric interaction with nearby materials, such as detector shielding, can produce characteristic K x-rays from the shielding material. In the case of lead shielding these K x-rays lie in the energy range of 72–88 keV (NIST 2020). However, these lead peaks are not always seen in practice (see figure 10.6).

5. *X-ray escape peak:* a characteristic x-ray may be produced following the photoelectric absorption corresponding to the K x-ray of iodine (28 keV). In most cases the x-ray is reabsorbed; however, if the photoelectric absorption occurs near the surface region, the x-ray can escape, which results in a decrease of the deposited energy. This x-ray escape peak is most likely to be observed with lower-energy gamma rays since, in this case, most events occur close to the surface of the crystal.
6. *Summation peak (true coincidence):* if radionuclides emit two gamma rays from the same disintegration, a coincidence or summation peak may occur. This peak corresponds to the sum of the gamma-ray energies and arises because of the simultaneous absorption of both gamma rays in the scintillator. Summation peaks are routinely used, for example, when counting ^{111}In or ^{125}I. These can additionally help to correct the counting efficiency, as described in section 6.8.
7. *Summation peak (random coincidence):* Summation peaks may also occur for radionuclides emitting monoenergetic gamma rays when there is a high count rate. When two gamma rays are emitted by different nuclei within the time resolution of the electronic detection system (random coincidence), they result in a single event with a summed energy. The probability of random coincidence increases as the count rate increases. This summation peak leads to loss of events for individual gamma-ray responses at high count rates. These can be corrected for, as described in section 2.5.2., although samples can ideally be diluted or left to decay before counting to reduce count losses due to random coincidences. Alternatively, some modern counters have a high-count-rate mode, which uses a robotic arm to lift the sample partly off the well to reduce counting efficiency and therefore random coincidences.

1.3.4 Energy resolution

When a NaI(Tl) detector is exposed to a monoenergetic beam of gamma rays, all photoelectric events (except for a few in which the iodine x-ray escapes) have the same energy loss in the detector. However, as can be seen from figure 1.2, the photopeak comprises of a spread of pulse sizes. This results from random variations in the various energy conversion steps in the detection process. The width of the peak is primarily determined by the statistical variation in the number of photoelectrons produced at the photocathode of the PMT. The energy resolution is usually measured using the full width at half maximum (FWHM) of the photopeak and is often expressed as a fraction of the photopeak energy. For ^{137}Cs the energy resolution of the 662 keV peak is typically about 7% (i.e. the FWHM is ~45keV). As the resolution is statistically limited, it improves with increasing gamma-ray energy proportional to $1/E^{1/2}$. The relatively good energy resolution of NaI(Tl) detectors means that it is possible to count samples containing a mixture of more than one radionuclide by using dual energy window counting and making appropriate correction for crosstalk between channels (section 9.7).

1.3.5 Counting efficiency

The counting of a sample is achieved by setting an appropriate pulse size window, which is often centered around the photopeak of the spectrum of the radionuclide. The counting efficiency (*E*) is defined as:

$$E = \frac{c}{d} \times 100$$

where *c* is the number of counts per second detected and *d* is the number of disintegrations per second in the sample. It depends on several factors, which can be described by the following equation:

$$E = A \cdot G \cdot D \cdot W \cdot (1 - S)$$

where *A* is the abundance of gamma photon production by the radionuclide, *G* is the geometric efficiency of photon detection, *D* is the intrinsic efficiency of the detector, *W* is the fraction of counts detected in the selected energy window, and S is the fraction of photons attenuated in the sample or vial wall.

The geometric efficiency is maximised by surrounding the sample as completely as possible with the detector. Fortunately, NaI(Tl) can be machined into a variety of shapes; those most commonly used are a well, first described by Anger (1951), and a diametric through hole (see figure 1.3), both of which give a geometric efficiency of almost 100 % with small volume samples. However, geometric efficiency is very dependent on the sample volume, particularly if activity extends near to or beyond

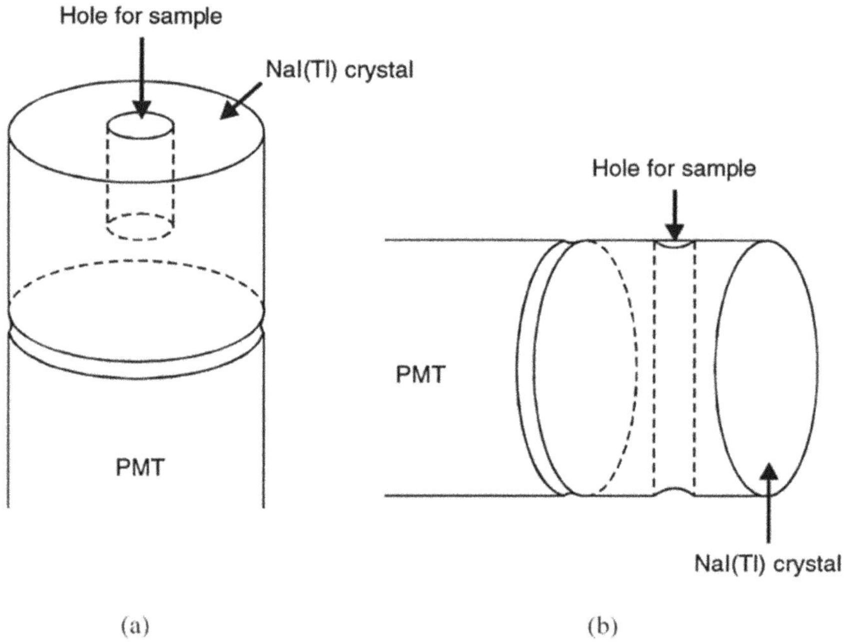

Figure 1.3. NaI(Tl) detectors: (a) well-type; (b) diametric through-hole type.

the edge of the detector, and this must be taken into consideration when carrying out measurements (see section 4.6.13 for sample volume effects).

The size of the sample also influences the self-absorption fraction, *S*. This effect is more marked for low-energy emitters such as ^{125}I (with energy peaks at 27 keV and 35.5 keV). For a particular application, the use of a constant sample volume and shape ensures that the geometric efficiency remains fixed. The intrinsic efficiency, *D*, is defined as the ratio of the number of pulses interacting in the detector to the number of gamma-ray photons which enter it. It increases with increasing crystal size and decreasing gamma-ray energy (figure 1.4(a)). The intrinsic efficiency value is close to unity for gamma-ray energies of less than 200 keV and medium-sized crystals.

The counting efficiency is also affected by the fraction of the detected spectrum which is used. It is common practice to eliminate rays scattered within the sample by counting only the photopeak, although in many applications this is not essential. Increasing the window width increases the relative contribution of background counts. If background contributions are substantial then a photopeak window should be used.

This is also the case when counting more than one radionuclide simultaneously. In this situation, the fractional detection in the window (W) is referred to as the photofraction, which is the fraction of the total number of pulses occurring in the spectrum that lie in the total energy peak. The photofraction increases with increasing crystal size and decreasing gamma-ray energy (figure 1.4(b)).

Typical counting efficiencies for commonly used radionuclides using a 3-inch diameter well-shaped crystal and an open energy window are shown in table 1.1.

Gamma counters are normally used to assay sample counts relative to counts for a standard. By relating the standard counts to a traceable absolute measure of activity, the counting efficiency can be determined and therefore the sample activity can be calculated.

1.4 Liquid scintillation counting

Liquid scintillation counting (LSC) uses a liquid scintillator to convert energy from nuclear emissions into light photons which are detected by PMTs. The scintillator is known as a liquid scintillation cocktail and comprises a solvent and several solutes (often referred to as scintillants, fluors, or lumiphors); it is usually dispensed into a glass or plastic vial before the addition of a radioactive component. The vial is placed into a light-tight chamber known as a light guide, which is connected to (typically) two PMTs, and a spectral output is recorded. Liquid scintillation counting is very versatile, and the cocktail choice allows the efficiency to be optimised for both the chemistry of the radioactive component and the emission type. Typically, liquid scintillation cocktails are optimised to provide high counting efficiencies for alpha and beta emissions from liquid radioactive samples (often with weak acidic or basic chemistries); however, solid samples and other emission types are also commonly counted using this method. A detailed description of the physical principles and practical considerations of liquid scintillation counting is provided in chapter 6.

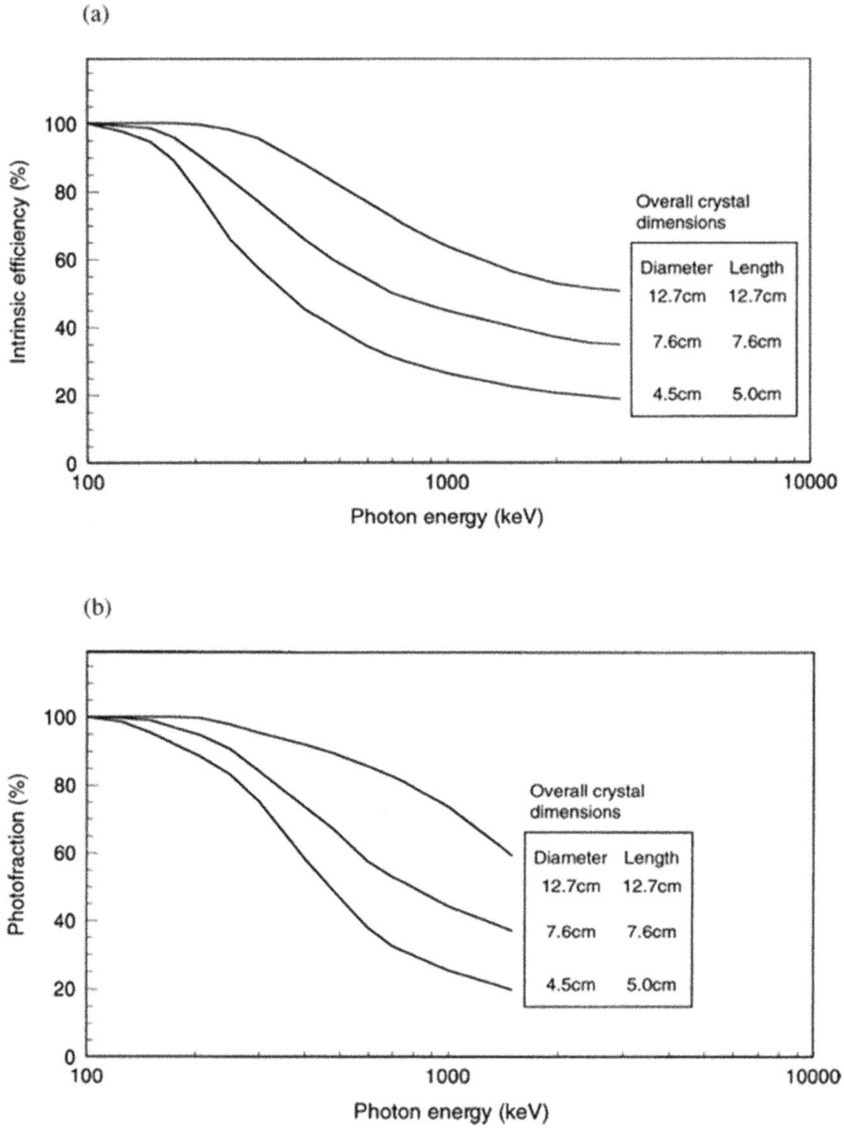

Figure 1.4. The variation of (a) intrinsic efficiency and (b) photofraction with energy for well-shaped NaI(Tl) crystals of varying size.

1.5 Solid-state detectors

Solid-state detectors are increasingly being used in nuclear medicine and health physics applications. Solid-state detectors, also known as semiconductor detectors, are made of solid materials with a crystalline structure. This crystalline structure has bandgaps of a few electron volts (eV). The majority of electrons in semiconductor materials are bound to specific sites in the lattice of the crystal within a low-energy state described as the valence band. When radiation is absorbed by a solid-state

Table 1.1. Counting efficiencies for some commonly used gamma-emitting radionuclides using a 76 mm long, 76 mm diameter well-type sodium iodide (Tl) detector with an open energy window.

Radionuclide	Principal gamma energy (keV)	Efficiency (%)
^{125}I	29	82
^{99m}Tc	140	89
^{123}I	159	89
^{131}I	364	43
^{58}Co	810	65
^{59}Fe	1292	28

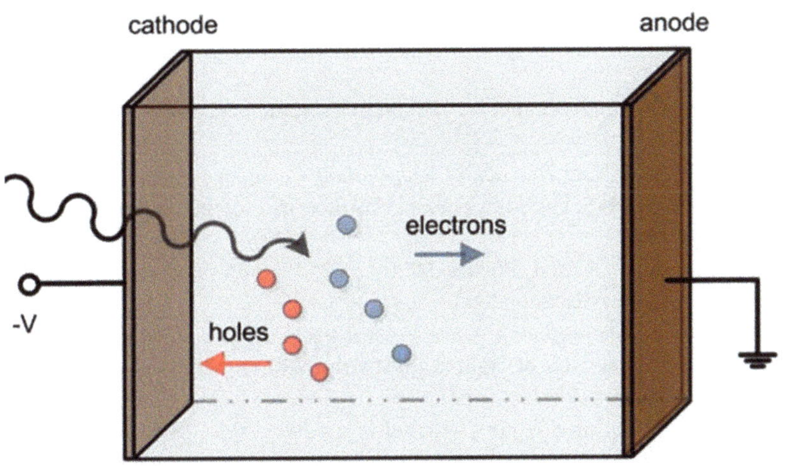

Figure 1.5. Planar configuration of a semiconductor detector. A voltage is applied between cathode and anode. As radiation interacts with the detector material, electron–hole pairs are created, which drift as a result of the voltage, creating an electric pulse. Reproduced under the Creative Commons license (Zhang *et al* 2013).

detector, ionisation occurs, which moves bound electrons out of the valence band and into a conduction band. In this high-energy state, the conduction electrons can flow freely, similarly to electrons in a metal. The vacancies left behind by excited electrons are known as holes, and they behave as positive charge carriers. Under the influence of an electric field, free electrons and holes drift in opposite directions towards opposite electrodes in the detector's surface, as shown in figure 1.5, generating an electric pulse.

When radiation interacts with a semiconductor material, the number of electron–hole pairs formed is proportional to the radiation energy absorbed, which is, in turn, proportional to the amplitude of the electric pulse generated.

Certain semiconductor materials, such as germanium or silicon-based materials, need to operate in low temperatures (i.e. −196 °C), to suppress the formation of electron–hole pairs due to thermal vibrations. These operating conditions are not practical for most clinical applications. Instead, semiconductor materials with wide bandgaps are used clinically, as they can operate at room temperature without the need for cooling devices (Cherry *et al* 2012).

One such material is cadmium zinc telluride (CZT). This is a compound semiconductor with a high density and a high effective atomic number, resulting in high detection efficiency (Takahashi and Watanabe 2001). The direct conversion of incident radiation into an electrical signal reduces statistical noise, producing superior energy resolution to that of scintillation detectors. However, due to the low mobility of charge carriers, the timing resolution of CZT is inferior to those of scintillation detectors, and in addition, the semiconductor material cost is relatively high (Zhang *et al* 2013).

CZT is frequently used in intraoperative probes, as its high efficiency facilitates the detection of low levels of radioactivity, while its excellent energy resolution enables scatter rejection.

References

Anger H O 1951 Scintillation counters for radioactive sample measurement *Rev. Sci. Instrum.* **22** 912–14

Birks J B 1964 *The Theory and Practice of Scintillation Counting* (Oxford: Elsevier)

Blau M and Dreyfus B 1945 The multiplier photo-tube in radioactive measurements *Rev. Sci. Instrum.* **16** 245–48

Cherry S R, Sorensen J A and Phelps M E 2012 *Physics in Nuclear Medicine* 4th edn (Philadelphia, PA: Elsevier Saunders)

Hine G J (ed) 1967 *Instrumentation in Nuclear Medicine* (Cambridge, MA: Academic Press)

Hofstadter R 1949 The detection of gamma-rays with thallium-activated sodium iodide crystals *Phys. Rev.* **75** 796–810

Kallmann H 1950 Scintillation counting with solutions *Phys. Rev.* **78** 621–22

NIST 2020 X-ray transition energies database (https://physics.nist.gov/cgi-bin/XrayTrans/search.pl?element=Pb&trans=All&lower=&upper=&units=eV)

Raben M S and Bloembergen N 1951 Determination of radioactivity by solution in a liquid scintillator *Science* **114** 363–64

Takahashi T and Watanabe S 2001 Recent progress in CdTe and CdZnTe detectors *IEEE Trans. Nucl. Sci.* **48** 950–59

Zanzonico P and Heller S 2000 The intraoperative gamma probe: basic principles and choices available *Semin. Nucl. Med.* **30** 33–48

Zhang Q *et al* 2013 Progress in the development of CdZnTe unipolar detectors for different anode geometries and data corrections *Sensors* **13** 2447–474

Chapter 2

Nucleonic equipment

Sofia Michopoulou

2.1 Introduction

The fundamental concepts of modern gamma and beta sample counters have changed little over the past 20 years. The main areas of advancement have been associated with signal digitisation, computerised online data acquisition, and analysis systems. However, the design of modern counters provides little insight into the structure of the underlying nucleonic equipment. It remains important to understand the influence of the component parts of this equipment on system stability, peak selection, and count-rate response. The main building blocks of gamma and beta detection systems are illustrated in figures 2.1 and 2.2, and these will be briefly reviewed in this chapter. More detailed descriptions can be found in Knoll (2010) and Cherry, Sorenson, and Phelps (2012).

2.1.1 Digital pulse processing

Traditionally, counting systems were made of analogue component chains, as shown in figure 2.2. Each component performed a specific function and when connected together they would provide all the measurements of interest. In the traditional setup, the analogue signal was amplified and shaped prior to digitisation.

Nowadays, digitisation takes place early on in the chain using fast and high-precision analogue-to-digital converters (ADCs). In this setup, the linear amplifier and analogue pulse-shaping circuits are replaced by a flash ADC and digital signal processors (DSPs), as shown in figure 2.3, which digitize and process pulses in real time (IAEA 2009, Tintori 2011).

Digital pulse processing offers a few advantages over analogue processing, including:

- improved energy resolution to the early signal digitisation and optimal noise suppression
- upgradable/reprogrammable logic
- adaptive pulse shaping, including improved pulse pile-up rejection

doi:10.1088/978-0-7503-3895-0ch2

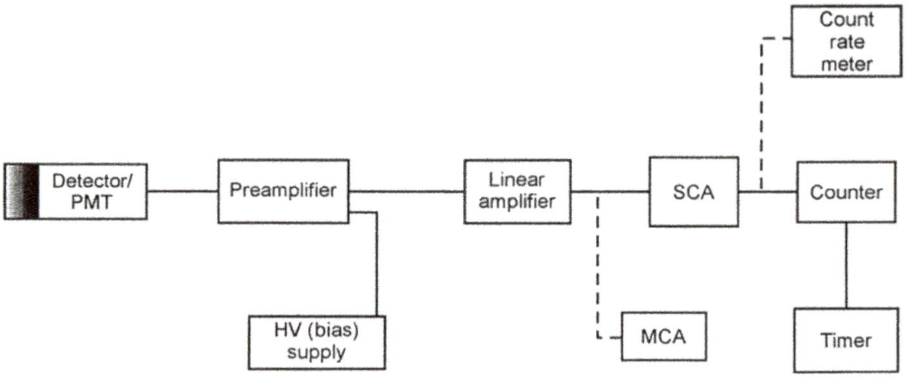

Figure 2.1. Solid scintillation detector system. *HV is the high-voltage supply, SCA is the single-channel analyser, and MCA is the multichannel analyser.

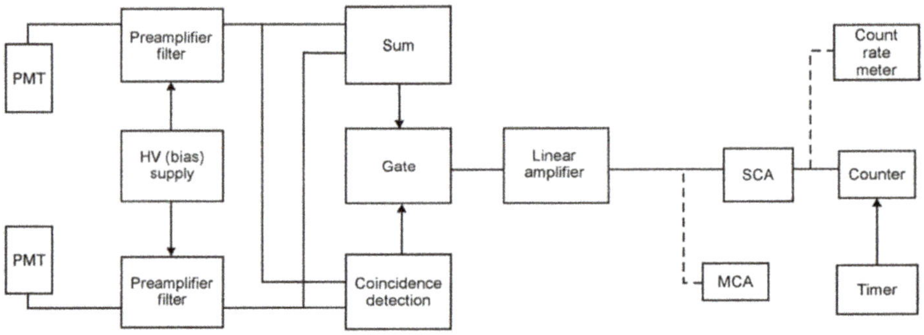

Figure 2.2. Liquid scintillation detector system.

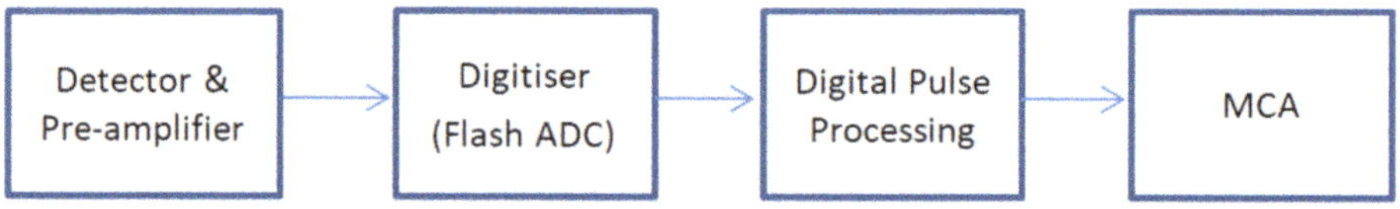

Figure 2.3. Counting system with digital pulse processing.

There are also a number of disadvantages of digital pulse processing compared to analogue techniques, including:

- limited amplitude precision due to quantisation
- stability issues arising from rounding errors

Further information on digital pulse processing is available in the International Atomic Energy Association's Technical Document 1634 (IAEA 2009). The remainder of this chapter will focus on describing the design and function of the key components used in sample counters.

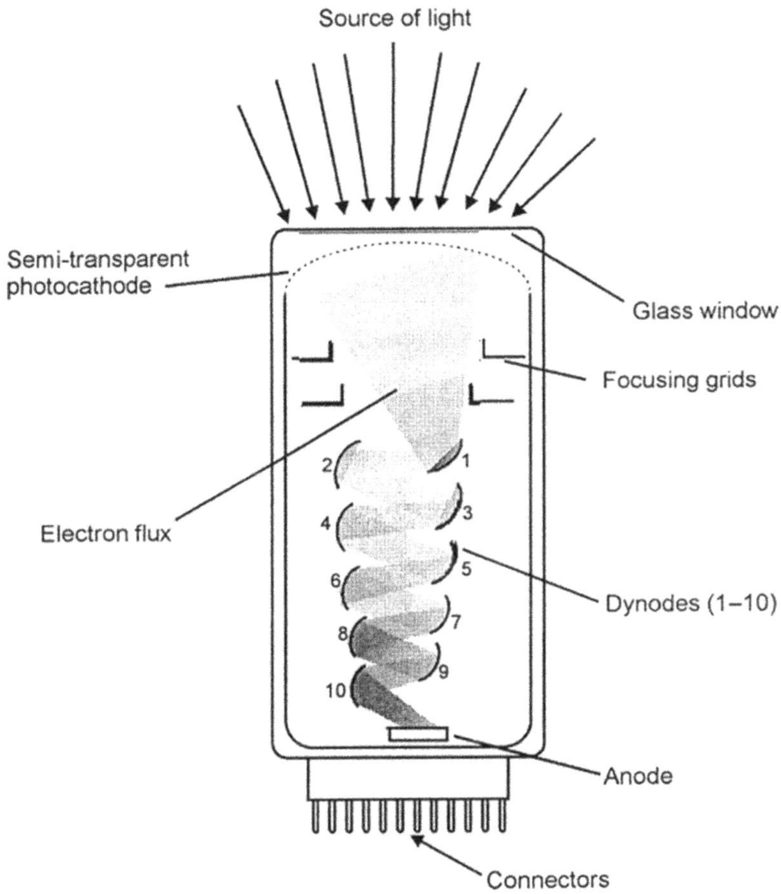

Figure 2.4. Structure of a PMT.

2.2 Photomultiplier tubes

Gamma and beta counter systems utilise solid and liquid scintillation detectors, respectively. The scintillation mechanisms differ, but each results in a detected event that produces a small amount of light. This light, typically ranging from a few hundred to a few thousand photons, is detected and converted into a usable electrical signal by a PMT. The PMT is an example of a vacuum tube, which is a very sensitive light detector. It consists of a photocathode and an electron multiplier structure, as illustrated in figure 2.4; this structure is examined in more detail below.

2.2.1 Photocathode

The inside surface of the glass window of a PMT is coated with a semi-transparent layer of a photoemissive substance, referred to as the photocathode. This releases electrons (photoelectrons) when struck by photons in the visible or near-visible range of the electromagnetic spectrum. Photoemission consists of the transfer of the photon energy to an electron, the movement of that electron to the surface of the photocathode, and the removal of the electron from the photocathode. The energy transferred to the photoelectron is given by the quantum energy of the photon $h\nu$, where h is Planck's constant and ν is the frequency of the photon.

However, as the photoelectron moves to the surface, some energy is lost, and to leave the surface, the photoelectron has to overcome a potential barrier (or work function) between the photocathode and vacuum. The energy of the photoelectron is given by:

$$(h\nu - W),$$

where W represents the work function of the photocathode.

The photocathode produces thermionic emissions and spontaneously induced electrons which constitute noise in the signal and are known as the dark current. Materials based on caesium–antimony (CsSb), referred to as bialkali, are suitable for photocathodes due to their high sensitivity and low thermionic emission. Ideally, the response of the photocathode should be optimal for the energy of the photons being detected. One way to express the sensitivity of a photocathode is by its quantum efficiency (QE). This is defined as:

$$QE = \frac{\text{number of photoelectrons emitted}}{\text{number of incident photons}}.$$

Quantum efficiencies of 20%–30% are obtainable with routinely used PMTs. Electrons from the photocathode are accelerated by an electric field and guided over a short distance by focusing grids to an electrode referred to as a dynode. This first dynode is held at a positive potential (200–300 V) above that of the photocathode.

2.2.2 Electron multiplier

Photoelectrons impacting the first dynode cause the excitation and subsequent emission of secondary electrons. The electrons are accelerated towards the second dynode in the chain, due to the positive potential between the dynodes. The impact of these electrons on the second dynode results in excitation and emission of further electrons. This process is repeated over ten to twelve dynode stages in a typical PMT. The number of secondary electrons released at each stage is a function of the dynode material and the incident electron energy and is typically five to ten secondary electrons. Considering that there are ten to twelve dynode stages, this results in a multiplication factor of 10^5–10^7 secondary electrons per photoelectron. Higher numbers of secondary electrons per stage can be achieved by negative electron affinity materials, such as zinc-doped gallium phosphide (GaP). An important feature of the PMT is the proportionality between the intensity of the light striking the photocathode and the output pulse size or amount of current produced.

2.2.3 Photomultiplier tube characteristics

PMTs are sealed glass tubes whose electrical contacts for the photocathode, focusing grids, dynodes, and anodes are made via pin connections in the base. They are usually enclosed in a 'mu-metal' alloy screen to remove the effect of external magnetic fields. Tubes used for scintillation counting have flat end windows matching the tube diameter. Various dynode configurations are available, namely, focused linear structure, circular grid, Venetian blind, and box and grid. Venetian blind and box and grid geometries represent older designs; linear structures and circular grids were introduced more recently to enable faster electron transit times through the tube. Some of the factors taken into consideration when manufacturers select a PMT specification include: the mean electron transit time and its distribution, maximum current and voltage ratings, dark current, linearity, photocathode non-uniformities, and gain variation with count rate.

Background current may arise from natural radioactivity within the tube structure, possible sources of which are radioactive potassium or thorium within the glass window. PMTs should never be exposed to ambient light when a high voltage is applied, as the anode current limit will be exceeded and damage will occur. Even without an applied voltage, exposure to ambient light, in particular, that of fluorescent tubes, is to be avoided. In spectrometry the performance of the PMT can play an important role in determining the energy resolution of the detector system.

2.3 High-voltage supply

Scintillation detectors incorporating a photomultiplier tube require a high-voltage (HV) supply, often referred to as the detector bias supply. The function of the HV supply is to ensure that the photocathode and succeeding dynode stages are correctly biased with respect to one another. Generally, the bias voltages at each stage are provided by a single supply distributed via a resistive voltage divider. The voltage across the photocathode and first dynode is usually two or three times greater than the interdynode potential. A typical interdynode potential is 100 V.

Stability is an important characteristic of an HV supply. The gain of the PMT is very sensitive to variations in applied voltage. Typically, a 1% change in HV will produce a 10% change in anode signal. HV supply characteristics detailing the change in output with respect to mains supply, temperature, time, and the degree of ripple are usually taken into consideration. A high-quality commercial HV supply will have a voltage output that is variable from 300–3000 V and a stability better than 0.01% per 10% change in mains voltage, 0.01% per hour (at constant mains voltage and temperature) and 0.02% per °C temperature variation.

2.4 Pulse amplifiers

Scintillation detectors produce discrete signal pulses with a short duration and an amplitude proportional to the energy of the incident radiation. The output from a NaI(Tl) scintillation detector is typically 0.5–2.0 V, with a pulse duration (mean decay time) of 250 ns. Corresponding figures for a liquid scintillation detector are

0.05–0.2 V and 10 ns. The role of the amplifier is to convert the detector output signal into a form compatible with subsequent pulse analysis modules (see figures 2.1 and 2.2).

Traditional detector systems operate using two amplifiers, the preamplifier and the linear (or main) amplifier. In newer digital systems, early digitisation is performed by a flash ADC, as shown in figure 2.3. Further details of detector design in relation to signal amplification and signal shaping are available in Knoll (2010), Tintori (2011) and Cherry, Sorenson, and Phelps (2012).

2.5 Pulse analysis and recording

The output from the amplifier stage of a scintillation detector is a succession of variable-amplitude pulses, in which the amplitude is proportional to the energy of the detected event. Restricting the pulse counting to a range of energies permits the events occurring due to background or scattered radiations or arising from system noise to be excluded. Examination of the energy signal in this manner is referred to as pulse height analysis.

2.5.1 Multichannel analyser

In modern counting systems, pulse height analysis is carried out by a multichannel analyser (MCA). The MCA uses a fast ADC to convert the incoming analogue pulses into a digital signal. The ADC sorts the pulses into bins (channels) according to their height (amplitude). Each channel corresponds to a certain energy range in the spectrum.

The MCA performs simultaneous recording of detected events in multiple energy windows to create a histogram (energy spectrum) and facilitate pulse height analysis. The range of pulse heights to be analysed can be selected by defining the upper and lower level discriminators of the energy window. The pulse height data are stored in digital memory and the address of each memory location corresponds to a channel. The output of the multichannel analyser is sent to the acquisition computer for storage, display, and analyses.

The ADC plays a major role in the overall performance of the MCA. Factors that influence its performance are: (a) conversion time, the time required to determine the digital representation of the analogue signal; (b) linearity, the relationship between the signal amplitudes and channel number; and (c) resolution (conversion gain), the number of digital bits into which the signal can be converted. An 8-bit ADC is able to identify 256 separate channels. Modern systems often offer over 2000 separate channels for pulse height analysis.

2.5.2 Dead time

Every counting system takes a finite time to process an individual detected event. During this time, the system will not respond correctly to any new events and, in consequence, it is referred to as the dead time. As radioactive decay in the sample is a random process, there is always a probability that for two events occurring in succession, the second will be lost because it enters the counting system too soon after the first. This is referred to as a dead-time loss, and such losses become severe when high count rates are encountered. Counting systems are considered to have either a paralysable or non-paralysable response. In non-paralysable systems, any event entering the detector during the dead-time window of the previous event is ignored. For this reason, with an increasing event rate, the detector will reach a saturation rate. The true count rate (R_t) for non-paralysable systems is given by:

$$R_t = \frac{R_0}{1 - R_0\tau},$$

where R_0 is the observed count rate and τ the system dead time.

In paralysable systems, the dead time is extended by a further period of the system dead time for every subsequent event entering the detector. For paralysable systems the relationship is given by:

$$R_0 = R_t e^{-R_t\tau}.$$

In this case there is no explicit solution for the true count rate (R_t). However, for low true count rates ($R_t \ll 1/\tau$), both non-paralysable and paralysable systems approximate to:

$$R_0 = R_t(1 - R_t\tau).$$

For a non-paralysable system the observed count rate can rise to a maximum limit and remain there, irrespective of any further increase in the true count rate. A paralysable system will display a maximum observed count-rate limit, but on a further increase in the true count rate, the observed rate will reduce and eventually approach zero.

Detector systems incorporating an MCA have dead-times in the order of 10 μs or more. This time is dominated by the ADC conversion and memory storage times. MCAs have the ability to correct the acquisition time to account for the losses due to dead time. This is referred to as 'live-time' counting and is relatively accurate provided that the fractional loss does not exceed 30%–40%. When designing a counting protocol it is important to ensure that the levels of activity in the sample are within a range that minimises dead-time losses to improve counting accuracy. Dilution of samples or a delay and decay approach can be used to ensure that dead-time losses are sufficiently low. System dead-time and count-rate performance at high activities should be assessed during commissioning, as outlined in section 4.6.12.

References

Cherry S R, Sorensen J A and Phelps M E 2012 *Physics in Nuclear Medicine* 4th edn (Philadelphia: Elsevier Saunders)

IAEA 2009 Signal processing and electronics for nuclear spectrometry 2007. IAEA-TECDOC-1634, Vienna

Knoll G 2010 *Radiation Detection and Measurement* 4th edn (New York: Wiley)

Tintori C 2011 *Digital pulse processing in nuclear physics* WP2081 1–21 CAEN S.p.A. white paper

IOP Publishing

Radioactive Sample Counting: Principles and Practice (Second Edition)
IPEM report 85
Sofia Michopoulou

Chapter 3

Quality control charts

Andrew Fenwick

3.1 Introduction

Quality control charts are primarily a visual tool that can be used to identify trends and outliers in a measured dataset. The goal is to identify a statistical process and monitor it over time to recognise variations from this process (outside the typical expected statistical variance) using control limits. Control charts can quickly show whether an item of equipment is drifting from its normal operation and requires maintenance or recalibration, and they give a visual representation of the equipment's performance over time, enabling the operator to identify trends which may indicate an impending problem. The control chart used is dependent on the nature of the process being monitored and therefore multiple charts may be used for a single item of equipment, depending on the critical processes being observed. There are vast number of different control charts, which are discussed at length in the standard ISO 7870 (ISO 2019); however, three of the most relevant control charts for use with radioactive counting equipment are summarised here. Each piece of radioactive counting equipment should have some form of control chart if it is used for routine work, and any site that has (or is seeking) accreditation should take particular care to ensure that its control charts are appropriate and are regularly updated.

3.2 Types of control chart

This chapter focusses on three main types of control chart which are frequently used with radioactive sample counting equipment. This is not an exhaustive list, and readers should consult ISO 7870 or the equipment manufacturer to ensure that the correct charts are being used for their equipment. The majority of the equipment used in a clinical environment can be monitored using one of the charts described below:

a) **Shewhart Control Chart**—This control chart is used to identify variations in a dataset that are not due to normal statistical variation. The chart comprises a dataset plotted between control limits which are determined using a representative dataset which is deemed to be the control. If measurements fall outside the control limits, then the reasons for this should be investigated before work continues. This chart monitors the long-term stability of a process; however, it can also be used as part of acceptance testing with a smaller dataset. These charts can be used to monitor the stability of most radioactive counting equipment. This chart type is discussed in detail in BS ISO 7870–2:2013 (ISO 2013).

b) **CUSUM Control Chart**—The CUSUM (cumulative sum of differences) chart is used to identify trends in datasets more readily. Plotting the difference between measurements makes it quite apparent when trends begin to emerge, and the CUSUM chart can be useful in identifying when a change occurred in order to help identify the reason for the variation. A CUSUM chart is typically used in conjunction with another control chart (such as a Shewhart chart) as an additional indicator of equipment performance and to aid in identifying the causes of issues. This chart is discussed in detail in BS ISO 7870:4:2011 and BS 5703:2011 (ISO 2011).
c) **Trend Control Chart**—The trend control chart monitors a process that is known to change over time as the result of a non-statistical process. For these systems, a Shewhart chart becomes ineffective because, from a mathematical perspective, the measurements are not strictly governed by a statistical process, but there is an underlying stochastic process that must be considered. By establishing the known trend in a process, control limits can be applied such that a larger or smaller drift is quickly identified and can be investigated. This chart type is discussed in detail in BS ISO 7870–5:2014 (ISO 2014).

Most radioactive counting equipment can be effectively monitored using Shewhart and CUSUM control charts, and therefore worked examples of these can be found in section 10.10.

3.3 Shewhart control chart

To create a Shewhart control chart, the user must first identify the baseline characteristics of the system they want to monitor. For instance, tracking the observed count rate response of a gamma counter to a standard source provides an indication of system stability. To construct a control chart, a routine measurement protocol can be established that involves measurements of a long-lived radioactive check source (such as ^{137}Cs) performed at a suitable frequency. Once a baseline has been established (such as taking 20 measurements), an average count rate ($\bar{X}$) can be determined using the values (decay corrected to a common reference time) and an associated standard deviation (σ). This information can then be used to determine some control boundaries at $\bar{X} \pm 2\sigma$ and $\bar{X} \pm 3\sigma$, which represent 'warning' and 'control' limits, respectively. By plotting a graph as shown in figure 3.1, the performance of the system can be visually tracked and action taken if measurements fall outside the warning or control limits. It is important that new measurements do not alter the established control limits, and should the system undergo a systematic

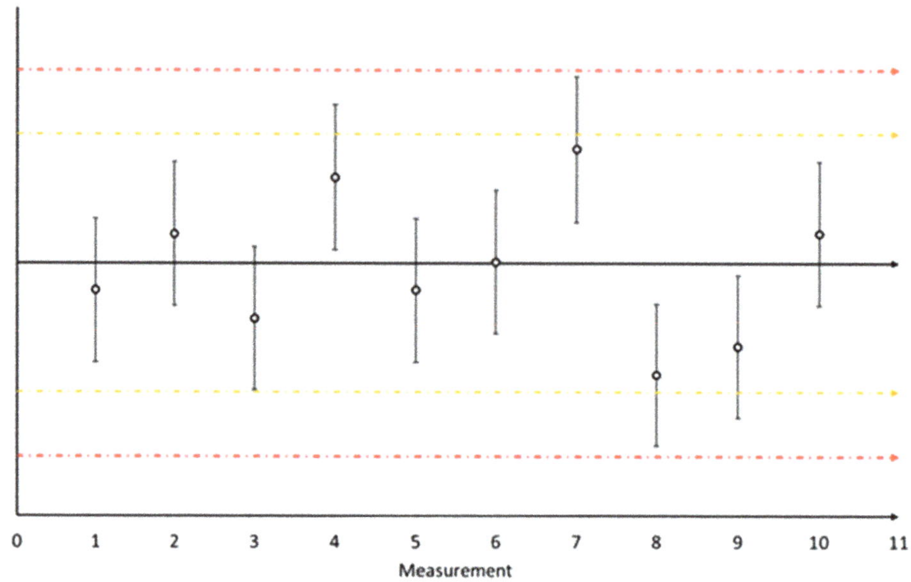

Figure 3.1. An example of a Shewhart Chart depicting warning (yellow line) and control (red line) limits determined using the statistical variation of the input data. The central black line indicates the mean of the control dataset. The error bars are determined by calculating the statistical error of the measurement.

change then the process must be restarted, and new limits determined. Other trends which may be useful to note would be a series of points above or below the average, or a series of increasing or decreasing points, as both of these can indicate that the system has deviated from normal statistical control and may require attention soon.

A variation to this form of chart is to use a reference value obtained from a calibration certificate and apply limits according to performance requirements. This involves applying a fixed control limit, which is not based on the dataset itself, but based on some other factor, such as user performance requirements. These charts may help if the process includes some stochastic effects that are difficult to capture in other ways (such as weighing errors or equipment linearity). Care should be taken when using such a chart, as limits can become significantly greater than the statistical variation of the subset and problems with equipment may not be identified until a critical failure has occurred.

3.4 CUSUM control chart

The CUSUM control chart uses the same data as that for the Shewhart chart. However, instead of tracking the individual differences independently, each successive difference is summed, and the resulting cumulative sum is plotted in a sequential fashion, regardless of time interval. This allows the user to visually identify a trend emerging from the data, such as a series of increases or decreases which could indicate impending failure. The chart can also be used following a failure to identify when the problem began (e.g. when a system became contaminated during routine use).

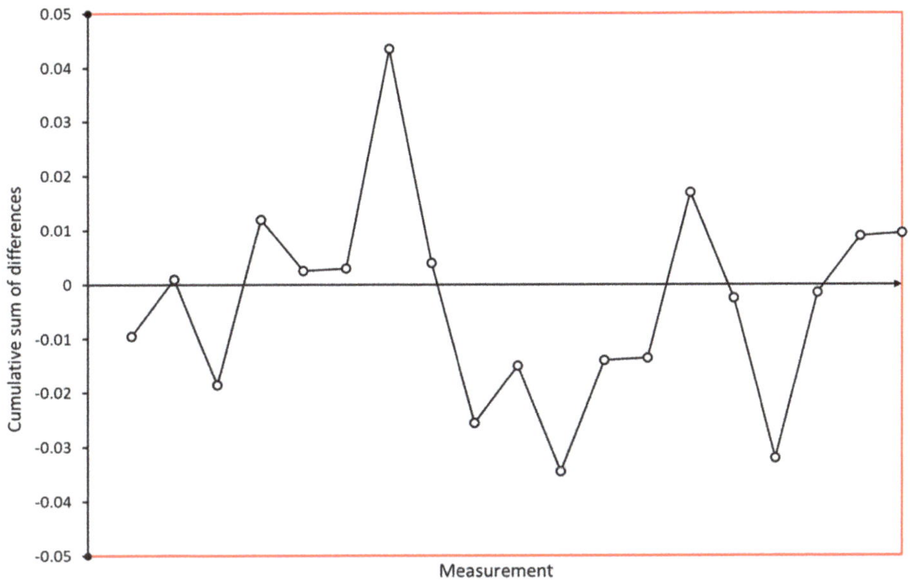

Figure 3.2. An example of a CUSUM control chart. The black line indicates the mean of a dataset, and the y-axis is fixed at 3σ to highlight a significant drift in the measured data.

To construct a CUSUM chart, a reference value must be identified (typically the mean of a measured dataset) and the difference of each measurement from the reference value is determined. These are progressively summed and plotted on a chart using an x-axis of equally spaced, arbitrary units to give a good visual effect (figure 3.2). Since the CUSUM chart is based on visual interpretation, it is important to fix the y-axis at a predefined limit so that it is easy to observe whether the system is operating correctly. This limit is dependent on the equipment in use. A recommended starting point is $\pm\ 3\sigma$, as consistent drifts greater than this in one direction indicate a drift in the mean of the dataset and are likely to highlight an instability in the system. Each CUSUM point $((Cu_X))$ is calculated by adding the difference $(X - \overline{X})$ to the previous CUSUM point $(Cu_{(X-1)})$, as shown in equation (3.1):

$$Cu_X = Cu_{(X-1)} + (X - \overline{X}). \tag{3.1}$$

3.5 Trend control chart

The trend control chart monitors systematic change within a system. In the case of radioactive sample counters, the principal application of this chart type would be to monitor the efficiency of ^{14}C or tritium standards in a liquid scintillation counting system. The PMTs used in liquid scintillation counters degrade over time and therefore the efficiency observed also drops as the system ages. This drift is to be expected and should progress at a nominally steady rate; therefore, the trend control chart can be used to identify whether sudden changes of range have occurred between measurements, which would indicate a potential problem with the system (figure 3.3).

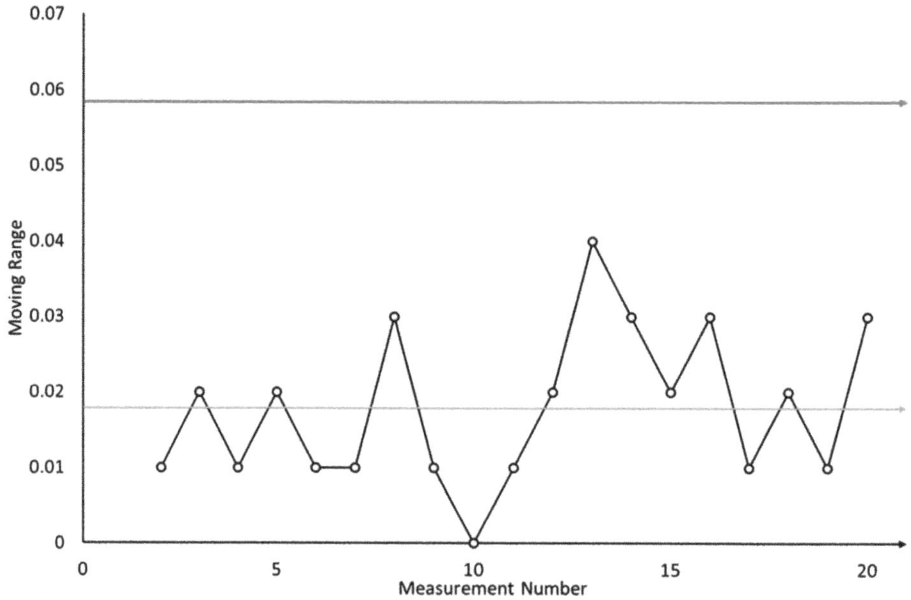

Figure 3.3. Trend control chart showing the measurement ranges observed plotted against the mean range (green line) and control range (red line).

To construct a trend control chart, it is important to first identify the typical 'drift' to be expected within the system. This may be provided by the manufacturer; however, it is common to determine this range using an existing dataset by calculating the difference between a subset of successive measurements and taking a mean. Limits may be set by multiplying this range by a suitable factor, depending on the performance expected of the system. It may be important to consider the time difference as well as device usage between measurements when using a range chart. Some systems may 'wear' in such a way that repeated measurements degrade the counting system, whereas others will 'age' regardless of the number and type of measurements taking place.

References

ISO 2011 BS ISO 7870-4:2011, control charts part 4: cumulative sum charts. BSI Standards Limited

ISO 2013 Control charts part 2: Shewhart control charts, ISO 7870-2:2013. ISO, International Organization for Standardization

ISO 2014 BS ISO 7870-5:2014, control charts part 5: specialized control charts. BSI Standards Limited 2014

ISO 2019 BS ISO 7870-1:2019 control charts, part 1: general guidelines. BSI, The British Standards Institution, 2019

IOP Publishing

Radioactive Sample Counting: Principles and Practice
(Second Edition)
IPEM report 85
Sofia Michopoulou

Chapter 4

Gamma counters

Lucy Pike and Fergus McKiddie

4.1 Introduction to gamma counter instrumentation

Automatic gamma counters have common basic features, as shown in figure 4.1. The integrated photomultiplier assembly is a sealed unit housing the sodium iodide crystal(s) and photomultiplier tube(s) and is a sealed unit. Commercially available gamma counters generally have a single well-type detector, which is suitable for small sample volumes and low-energy radionuclides such as ^{125}I, ^{57}Co and ^{99m}Tc. The detector chamber/photomultiplier assembly is shielded from external radiation sources, such as room background and other samples in the counter awaiting counting or having been counted, by typically >30 mm of lead shielding.

In gamma counters the sample may be loaded using a pick-up arm to lift the sample from the rack or belt of the sample transport system, and then lowered into the detector well in the crystal using a tube carrier. This method is suitable for use with a range of different sample vial sizes. The counting and the processing parameters are generally controlled via a touch screen control panel or online computer. Some gamma counters are now available with an optional integral balance for sample weighing to allow streamlined workflows.

The choice of vial is dependent on the application. The samples to be counted are typically contained in counting vials made of plastic. The range of vial sizes which can be used is dictated by the design of the specific sample counter, but the vials generally have a volume of less than 20 mL. Many gamma counters now allow the use of centrifuge tubes, which may reduce the number of sample transfers required.

Data counter results are accessible through a variety of output devices. The output may be directly sent to a printer, integral computer and printer, or via a Universal Serial Bus (USB) or ethernet connection to external devices. Integral computers can be networked to sample preparation systems, other counting equipment, or external computers. They also provide data storage, usually on internal hard drives. Real-time and retrospective quality control (QC) analysis is available with integral computer systems. QC measures can be

doi:10.1088/978-0-7503-3895-0ch4

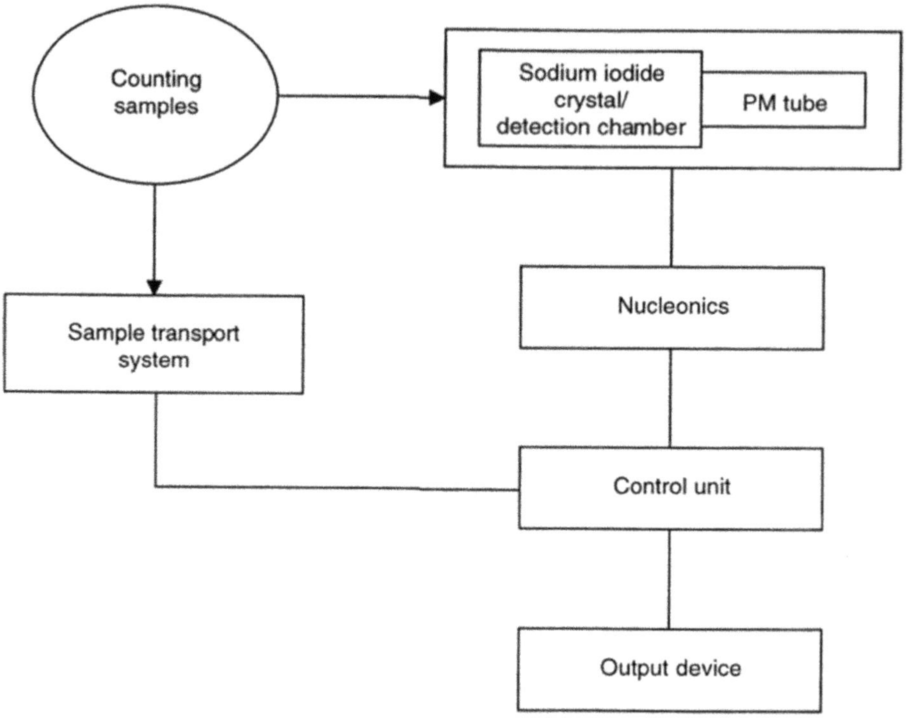

Figure 4.1. Basic features of a radioactive sample counter.

displayed graphically against time so that any systematic trends or large random deviations can be seen easily. Integral computers can allow the use of manufacturer-supplied software, the user's own software, and standard spreadsheets and databases.

4.2 Applications of gamma counters

Gamma counters are used in a range of clinical, research, and radiation safety applications, including:

- radioimmunoassay
- assessment of glomerular filtration rate
- measurement of blood and urine excretion rates for radionuclide dosimetry
- quality control of radioactive compounds to assess binding efficiency
- leak testing of sealed sources and wipe testing of surfaces

Practical worked examples of the clinical and research applications of gamma counters are outlined in chapter 10.

4.3 Gamma counter types

4.3.1 Multi-detector systems

Systems with multiple detector wells enable the simultaneous counting of up to 12 samples. These systems provide high throughput, which is essential for certain clinical applications that require an urgent report of counting results. Additionally, multi-detector systems are useful in counting radionuclides with short half-lives, as they enable simultaneous counting of multiple samples to avoid loss of counts due to decay.

The choice of single or multi-detector system depends on local requirements, as outlined in the procurement section 4.5. Multi-detector systems require detector response normalisation to ensure that equivalent readings are obtained from the different detector wells. This forms part of the routine quality control for these systems, as outlined in section 4.6.

4.3.2 Through-hole systems

In these systems, as shown in figure 1.3, the detector well is replaced by a hollow cylinder, open at the top and bottom surfaces. Through-hole systems have slightly lower efficiency than well systems of the same size. In through-hole crystals, samples are delivered to the sample changer and then elevated or dropped into position without a tube carrier, to reduce contamination risk. The sample changer can centre the sample within the detector, which compensates in part for differing sample sizes and reduces volume dependence, as discussed in section 4.6.13.

4.3.3 Gamma counters for PET radionuclides

Most gamma counter systems are designed to count low-energy emitters. Requirements for gamma counters for PET applications differ, due to the higher energy of the annihilation photons (511 keV). Gamma counters used for PET applications should ideally have a thicker NaI(Tl) crystal, providing increased detector efficiency. Additionally, thicker shielding is required between detectors for multi-detector systems and also between the detector and other samples in the counter (Lodge *et al* 2015).

Gamma counters are used in PET applications such as blood counting to calculate the arterial input function and to measure ^{68}Ge generator breakthrough, as outlined in chapter 10.

4.3.4 Sample transport systems

Automatic counters must be capable of handling a large number of possibly different types of sample vial in a rapid and efficient manner. The time taken to unload one sample from the detection chamber and load the next should be short but constant, to allow for decay correction when counting isotopes of very short half-life. Counters are available which can accommodate up to 1000 samples using multiple detectors and rack loading systems. Counters may have ‘sample present’ sensors to bypass empty sample vial positions. Electric motors are used to drive the sample transport system.

4.3.5 Rack-loaded systems

Individual batches of samples can be loaded on the bench into racks or cassettes with a capacity of 5–20 samples. Different sizes of rack/cassette are usually available to accommodate different vial sizes and special adapters are available for unusually short sample tubes. Racks can be loaded quickly and easily and may be used as sample carriers or during sample preparation in conjunction with an automatic pipetting station. Racks can be easily loaded, removed, or rearranged to accommodate changes in counting priorities. Sample cassettes may be transported on paired conveyor belts, one pair for right-to-left motion and one for the reverse. The sample changer is under microprocessor control and retractable drive pins move the cassette into the counting position or onto the other pair of belts once counting is completed. Well-type detector systems use a robotic lifting arm to lift the sample from the rack and then lower it into the well in the crystal using a tube carrier. Some counters additionally include an integral weight balance. This enables the individual samples to be weighed, which is particularly useful for certain clinical applications, such as the calculation of the glomerular filtration rate, as outlined in section 10.2.

4.4 Counting options

The different specific requirements of individual users of a gamma counter necessitate the facility to program counting sequences. The degree to which automatic collection and processing of sample data is available depends on the particular sample counter, although most now default to automatic operation with an option to switch to manual operation. Automation can range from manual selection of count, time, energy window, and background subtraction, to systems in which pre-set parameters are selected by the sample batches to control data handling with output via a computer. Automatic assay procedures in sample counters are generally now initiated by program selectors placed on the front of a rack which identify particular samples or batches of samples. The main features of the automatic programmed counting methods are described below.

4.4.1 Manual pre-selection

In the manual operation mode of modern counters, the sample count and/or time may be pre-set from the video display unit or the control console. Sample counts of up to about 100 kcts and times of up to 100 min are usually available. When either the pre-set count or time limit is reached, the counter automatically advances to the next sample. Another parameter which can be manually selected is the energy window. In addition to variable energy and window controls, pre-set values for a number of isotopes may be selected from the menu.

4.4.2 Programmable racks

In rack-loaded automatic counters, multi-purpose control may be effected by a coded strip, or barcode attached to a clip which fits on the outside of the sample rack. The barcode is sensed by an optical reader that identifies the rack so that counting and/or processing parameters are set using the encoded information to automatically select the energy channel, sample standardisation, counting time, computer analysis, and output format. The barcode therefore gives the counter complete instructions regarding the counting and processing of all samples in the batch preceded by the same barcode. Energy channels, or windows, are typically available for up to 99 pre-programmed isotopes or may be set by the user, for example if asymmetric windows are required. On PerkinElmer Wizard systems, barcodes are also available for functions such as efficiency normalization, background normalization, instrument performance assessment, and cessation of counting (PerkinElmer 2002). HIDEX systems also have automatic QC and daily stability settings to ensure consistency of performance (HIDEX 2017). Multiple label samples may also be counted for up to six isotopes simultaneously, although dual label operation is typically more likely. To achieve this, normalization must be carried out with the pair of isotopes to be counted to allow for the calculation of spillover correction.

4.4.3 Fixed versus dynamic window

When counting samples of a known isotope, a counting window is usually set to determine the lower and upper limits of the energies to be counted. This is typically centred around the photopeak. In order to determine the counting window boundaries in terms of MCA channels, a conversion factor (in keV/MCA channels) is used. The conversion factor can either use the 'nominal gain', which is a fixed value set by the vendor based on the optimal performance of the detectors and is the same irrespective of the isotope used, or an isotope-specific 'effective gain' can be used. The effective gain is determined by dividing the energy of the photopeak for the specific isotope (in keV) by the MCA channel measured for the photopeak during the most recent assay or normalisation for that isotope. The idea is that by using the effective gain, drifts in detector performance over time can be accounted for.

The counting window settings that determine which gain is used are referred to as either a fixed or dynamic counting window and the user can choose which to apply per protocol. For the fixed window, the nominal gain is used and this means that the lower and upper limits for the counting window remain fixed regardless of whether there is any drift in the measured photopeak. For the dynamic counting window, the effective gain is used to determine the lower and upper boundaries of the counting window, so that they follow any drift in the photopeak for that specific isotope. The dynamic window can be set to use the photopeak measured during the most recent normalisation, thus accounting for longer-term drifts in the detector response. In addition, the dynamic window can be set to determine the effective gain from the photopeak measured during the assay itself. This latter option is designed to account for short-term changes in detector response caused by changes in room temperature or sample activity (PerkinElmer 2002).

In general, it is recommended to use a fixed window when counting unknown samples or multiple isotope samples or when using an open counting window. The use of a dynamic window using the effective gain calculated from the isotope normalisation can be helpful to correct for long-term drifts in the detectors. However, problems can arise when using a dynamic window based on the photopeak energy of the current measurement. Any unexpected peaks caused by contamination, background sources, etc. can result in the incorrect localisation of the photopeak, which will result in the incorrect counting window being set.

Therefore, if large temperature variations or wide-ranging sample activity levels are not expected then this mode may be switched off.

4.5 Specification and purchase of gamma counters

Prior to the purchase of any new laboratory or medical equipment, it is important to determine the range and type of work that will be performed as well as the projected workload of the system. This will ensure value for money and that the equipment is fit for purpose over the lifespan of the system.

This section provides general advice and considerations for the purchase of gamma counters to count *in vitro* samples. Advice should be sought from your institution's supplies or purchasing department on the procedures to follow when purchasing medical equipment. A pre-purchase questionnaire, such as the National Health Service (NHS) pre-acquisition questionnaire (NHS 2010) that covers regulatory compliance, such as CE marking and EC Directives, as well as product support, should be provided as part of equipment procurement.

4.5.1 Purchase of gamma counters

A gamma counter should be a highly reliable system capable of both high-volume routine clinical testing and low-volume, varied research applications. With a range of options available that differ in terms of detection method, detector geometry, sample transportation, and data processing and output, valuable time can be saved by giving careful thought to the system requirements before a purchase is made.

The requirements for an *in vitro* sample counter will be determined by several local factors, including the range and energies of radionuclides to be measured and the size and quantity of the samples themselves. Before a decision is reached, it is important to assess the type and range of work for which the counter will be used. The choice can be made easier by considering the following aspects of a sample counter.

4.5.2 The detection chamber

The purchaser will need to make two fundamental decisions. First, should the instrument be based on a single or a multiple detector system? Second, what is the preferred size and geometry of the detector?

The answer to the first question will depend upon the number of samples to be counted. A single detector system is less complicated, eliminates the issues of crosstalk and sensitivity variations between detectors, and is also cheaper. On the other hand, a multi-detector system is capable of measuring samples simultaneously and can provide results much quicker, which is important in time-sensitive clinical situations such as when calculating the glomerular filtration rate (GFR) for chemotherapy dose calculation or counting isotopes with short half-lives.

An estimate of the number of tests, number of samples required per test, and typical sample counting time can help to determine the appropriate number of detectors and whether a single- or multi-detector system is required.

As regards detector size and geometry, the well-type detector has a slightly higher efficiency (for point sources) than a through-hole detector of equal size, whilst the through-hole detector allows automatic sample changers to centre the sample within the detector, thus compensating in part for differing sample sizes. However, sample volume correction may be required for both counter types, as outlined in section 4.6.13. Generally it is not good practice to mix sample volumes or different test-tubes within a counting session, as volume specific corrections would be needed.

The efficiency of the detector depends upon the radionuclide being measured. If the counter is only to be used for assaying ^{125}I (35 keV) then the crystal need only be 10 mm thick. However, if higher-energy emitters such as ^{131}I (364 keV) or ^{18}F (511 keV) are also to be counted, the crystal should be at least 30 mm thick in order to have sufficient stopping power. Care must be taken when examining the specification of the counter. Crystals may be quoted as, for example, 75 mm × 75 mm with a well diameter of 25 mm. The effective thickness is therefore only 25 mm, limiting counting efficiency for radionuclides with energies of >300 keV.

The manufacturer should specify the counting efficiencies and energy resolution for the radionuclides that are expected to be used. Low counting efficiency results in longer counting times. The settings of the pulse height analyser used for efficiency measurements should be stated. The energy resolution is the full width half maximum (FWHM) of the photopeak spectrum obtained using a narrow analyser channel width and is usually expressed as a percentage of the photopeak energy. It is usually specified for ^{129}I, ^{57}Co, and/or ^{137}Cs. Its value is a function of the crystal size and photopeak energy.

If high-energy emitters are to be counted, then it is essential to consider whether there is sufficient shielding or software correction to reduce the effect of crosstalk to acceptable levels. Crosstalk can occur between samples counted simultaneously in multi-detector systems and also between the detector and samples queueing on the conveyor to be counted later.

Tracer kinetic studies in PET require the counting of blood and plasma samples taken shortly after radiotracer administration. These tend to contain relatively high-activity concentrations compared to samples containing metabolites, therefore the detector dead time should be minimal at these high activities to ensure that the count-rate performance is linear over the range of sample activities to be counted. Certain detector systems offer a high count-rate mode, which is well suited for blood and plasma counting soon after administration.

4.5.3 Sample transport and capacity

The method of sample transport may be a significant factor in choosing a counter. The cost and availability of the consumables (tubing, vials, racks etc.) should be checked, especially if a high throughput is expected. Racks (or trays/cassettes) can be used to hold the vials throughout the laboratory procedure and not just when loaded on the counter. If it is intended to use them in this way, thought should be given to the purchase of extra racks. If a conveyor system is used, it is helpful if the movement can be reversed, as this speeds up sample loading. It is essential that the sample capacity is adequate for the expected workload. It is possible to increase the capacity of some instruments at a later date. The range of sample vial sizes that can be used may be important if more than one counter or other apparatus with vial size restrictions is to be used.

4.5.4 Data management and software

As large volumes of raw data may be generated, consideration should be given to the format and storage of the output produced by the counter. Methods of long-term archival and retrieval of the counter output should comply with data protection and retention policies for clinical and/or research data.

Generally, systems are PC-based and employ proprietary software. The software should be able to perform all required tasks, or if specialist processing is required, there should be a reliable way to export raw data from the counter in a standard format such as .txt or .csv for further analysis. It is also worth checking the extent to which the user is able to interrogate the results for the purposes of troubleshooting.

The latest generation of gamma and liquid scintillation counters employ a PC-based multichannel analyser allowing full-spectrum analysis to be performed. Data transfer to other devices is made far easier if the output of the counter is in a standard form. Raw or semi-processed data may then be routed via a local area network (LAN) to a data management system for further analysis, e.g. for the calculation of the glomerular filtration rate, and subsequent archiving.

For equipment in pharmaceutical laboratory environments where Good Manufacturing Practice (GMP) regulations apply, any software systems involved in the processing of electronic data as part of GMP-related activities such as product quality, process control, or quality assurance are required to implement access controls, audit trails, validation, electronic signatures, and documentation. Some manufacturers of sample counters have software that fulfils these requirements, but users should check whether this is an extra cost and what it covers. Legal requirements in the US are covered by the Food and Drug Administration's Title 21 Code of Federal Regulations Part 11 and in the EU by Good Manufacturing Practice 'Annex 11: Computerized Systems' .

As part of the specification, consideration should also be given to the PC operating system utilised to make sure it is currently supported, to determine whether the supplier provides support for software updates, and whether anti-virus software is included or can be installed, particularly if the PC is connected to the LAN.

4.5.5 Site planning

Before purchase, attention should be paid to the environment where the instrument is to be housed. Any electrical, temperature, ventilation, relative humidity, and siting (e.g. direct sunlight) requirements should be checked with the manufacturer.

The size of the instrument may be a critical factor for site planning, particularly if installation is in a small area or in a congested laboratory. It should be remembered that it might be necessary to provide access to the rear of the instrument for servicing. If free space cannot be allowed around the instrument, then it should be mounted on castors. The load bearing capacity of the floor or bench must also be considered, since larger models can be >300 kg with the lead shielding in place. Some manufacturers sell custom benches designed to hold their counters, which may be more suitable than laboratory benching.

Ideally, the counter should be sited away from any radioactive sources other than those to be counted. The thickness of lead surrounding the detection chamber determines the background count rate, and hence can influence the effective sensitivity of the counter. A thickness of 70 mm of lead should be adequate in most laboratories unless high activities of high-energy gamma emitters are used nearby. It must be remembered that the shielding should be designed for the worst-case situation. If a high-energy source is moved past the laboratory once a week, it will increase the background for a short period. An erroneous count will therefore be obtained for the sample being counted at that time. This situation should be avoided, if possible, by careful consideration of the siting of the counter. Increased shielding between the detection chamber and samples in the transport system is necessary for gamma counting to prevent increases in the local background due to the samples on the counter. This shielding should be at least twice as thick as that in other directions.

The electrical power consumption of the system is unlikely to be important, although the quality of supply may be. Transient pulses in the supply can cause counters to interrupt their normal operating sequence or, if a computer is used, they can cause data corruption and an unwanted interruption in the program. A similar effect may occur if the supply is switched to an emergency generator. Drift in the supply voltage can result in changes in the gain of the nucleonic equipment (section 2.3). The quality of the electrical supply should be checked against the manufacturer's requirements. It may be possible to overcome mains fluctuations by using an uninterruptible power supply (UPS) system.

4.5.6 Calibration sources

Long-lived radioactive sources are required for routine quality control and calibration of the sample counter. The type and activity of the sources required should be checked with the manufacturer, as well as whether these will be supplied with the counter or need to be purchased separately. These sources will need to be stored in a secure location, and should be subject to wipe testing, in line with the Ionising Radiation Regulations, 2017. Consideration should be given to the holding and storage of sources under local Environmental Permitting Regulations. A worked example of wipe testing is provided in section 10.6.

For sites using the sample counter for PET studies, there is the additional option of purchasing an aliquot of the uniform ^{68}Ge cylinder used for routine testing of the PET scanner. This ^{68}Ge aliquot can then be used as part of the routine QC of the sample counter, but it will need to be replaced along with the uniform cylinder on an 18–24 month basis.

The cost of source replacement and disposal needs to be considered at an early stage, as this can be expensive, even for sources of low activity.

4.5.7 Training and servicing

All manufacturers provide a warranty, normally for one year. After the warranty period has expired, continuing support from the manufacturer may be provided by a service contract. Both the service contract and the warranty should be inspected to determine the frequency of planned preventive maintenance visits, whether some or all parts are included, and whether breakdowns are covered. It is difficult to assess the value of a service contract without knowledge of the number of service engineers employed, the location of the nearest engineer, and the average speed of response. It is important to try to consult existing users of shortlisted instruments to obtain an impression of the service provided. The purchaser should check whether any training in the operation and setup of the sample counter is included as part of the installation, and if so, what is covered. This may be particularly useful if an unfamiliar model is being purchased.

4.5.8 Life cycle

As part of the purchase of new equipment, consideration needs to be given to the whole life cycle of the equipment, including decommissioning and disposal according to the relevant disposal regulations, including the Waste Electrical and Electronic Equipment (WEEE) Directive. This should also cover decontamination of the equipment (for radiation and biological contaminants) and removal/disposal of radioactive sources. In particular, the NaI(Tl) crystal is considered toxic and must be disposed of via authorised disposal routes, and the lead in the shielding is considered a pollutant and must be recycled appropriately.

4.5.9 Installation and commissioning

In general, installation will be performed by an authorised representative of the sample counter supplier. Operator manuals should be supplied and operator training should be provided. Before handover, the engineer should set up the counter and perform functional and performance checks to make sure the counter is operating as expected. It is also essential at this stage to arrange for electrical safety testing according to local laboratory or hospital policies, to ensure compliance with the current regulations.

Additional commissioning checks should be made locally by the medical physics expert (MPE). These will ensure that the instrument meets the specifications of the manufacturer and will also allow baseline values to be set for ongoing QC. Parameters such as the warm-up time, peak energy drift, energy linearity, energy settings, resolving time, crystal energy resolution, sensitivity, count-rate response, and the functioning of the data processing and sample transport systems should be thoroughly investigated and recorded for future reference and to set tolerances for routine QC. Suggested methods for testing the equipment are given in section 4.6. Standard operating procedures covering routine QC testing and operation of the sample counter should be written as part of the local quality assurance system. A logbook or electronic record system should be set up from installation, which will provide a service history of the instrument together with the means of drawing any recurring faults to the attention of the service engineer.

4.5.10 Legislative considerations regarding the purchase and use of radioactive sample counters in clinical practice

Radioactive sample counters may be used clinically to measure patient samples for, amongst other things, the purpose of non-imaging diagnostic studies or as part of dosimetry for radionuclide therapeutic or imaging studies. They can contribute to clinical evaluation of the study, as would be the case for samples counted on a gamma counter during a GFR test, or evaluate the dose delivered in the case of dosimetry studies. In such applications they are within the scope of the Ionising Radiation (Medical Exposure) Regulations 2017 legislation, which 'apply to the exposure of ionising radiation in England and Wales and Scotland' to individuals, including patients.

As such, the following individuals and issues should be considered:

- Prior to purchase, an entitled MPE must contribute to the preparation of technical specifications for the equipment and installation design and subsequently the definition and performance of quality assurance of the equipment, together with the acceptance testing of the equipment.
- The employer must implement and maintain a quality assurance programme, including written procedures for the quality assurance of the equipment and its subsequent clinical use. They must also include the equipment on their equipment inventory. It is the employer's responsibility to ensure that the equipment is tested prior to first use and that it subsequently undergoes regular periodic performance testing as well as additional testing in the event of a maintenance procedure which may impact the equipment's performance.
- Entitled operators involved in the testing and use of the equipment must be adequately trained, the training must be recorded, and continuing education must be undertaken as required. Such training may include:
    - Contributing to the quality assurance of the equipment, for example how to undertake daily quality control testing as part of a full quality assurance programme, or
    - Contributing to its clinical use, for example how to ensure it has been set up using the correct counting protocol and with appropriately prepared samples.

Additional legislation that may have to be considered includes the Medical Device Regulations (MDR). In this case any in-house software used to calculate clinical results would need to satisfy the regulations. For many hospitals this could include spreadsheets or similar which use the counts from a gamma counter to calculate patient GFR test results. Additionally, gamma counters can be used for leak testing as outlined in section 10.6, which is regulated under the Ionising Radiation Regulations 2017.

4.6 Quality assurance

Gamma counters may be in use almost continually and a thorough quality assurance system should be implemented to ensure that large numbers of clinical test results are not rendered invalid due to faults remaining undetected over long periods of time.

It is important that routine calibration is carried out and monitored by the user. The counter should be covered by a service and maintenance contract with either the manufacturer or a third-party provider.

Changes to performance parameters may be an indicator of developing problems in the detector(s), nucleonics, control unit, or sample transport system. Regular QC tests are essential to guarantee continued optimal performance. Many modern sample counters include the automated QC checks necessary to ensure consistency over long periods. If pre-set automatic QC protocols are not available, then the quality control tests described in this section should be performed on a regular basis. A summary of the tests and suggested frequencies is given at the end of this section in table 4.1.

4.6.1 Cleaning and decontamination

Full cleaning of the sample counter is usually included within the preventative maintenance visit under the service contract; however, any accessible counter surfaces and the conveyor should be regularly wiped down and cleared of any debris to avoid contamination or dust build-up. The user manual should indicate safe cleaning practices and non-corrosive materials that can be used for cleaning. The frequency of cleaning will depend on how much the counter is used, but should be included in the routine laboratory cleaning schedule.

4.6.2 Functional checks

Before each use the general condition and functioning of the sample counter should be checked visually. For sites with high-volume counting, this would typically be performed every day prior to counting the first series of clinical samples. If the use of the sample counter is less frequent, functional checks can be performed less often.

1. Inspect cables for wear and tear, particularly where they are flexed.
2. Check for signs of spills/contamination.
3. Clear the conveyor and remove any foreign objects from inside the detector assembly.
4. Check for faulty indicator lamps.
5. If an optical cap reader is employed, check alignment and clean as required. Inspect caps for cracks, burrs, etc.
6. Carry out a visual inspection of the transport system and check for smooth transport of the samples. This can be performed while the QC samples are counted.

4.6.3 Background checks

At installation, the background radioactivity should be measured for each detector using an open energy window under normal conditions and an empty sample tube in the well. This is used to determine a baseline for expected background levels. An important consideration is that impurities in the surrounding materials, including lead and steel, may result in a higher perceived background at baseline.

Occasionally, samples may spill inside the detection chamber. If this happens the resulting additional counts will be added to all subsequent samples measured. Some

Table 4.1. Recommended quality control tests and frequencies for gamma counters.

Test	Suggested frequency
Cleaning and decontamination	Daily/weekly depending on use.
Functional checks	Prior to counting session.
Background checks	Baseline measured at commissioning. Prior to and after each counting session.
Sensitivity	Baseline measured at commissioning. Annually and after any repairs.
Constancy of sensitivity and long-term stability	Tolerances set at commissioning or after major upgrade. Constancy of sensitivity measured prior to counting session and long-term stability assessed quarterly
Energy resolution and photo-peak channels	Checked prior to counting session Re-calibration performed as part of detector normalisation.
Normalisation	At commissioning and quarterly (unless otherwise specified by the manufacturer).
Cross-calibration	At commissioning and quarterly after normalisation.
Repeatability	At commissioning and annually.
Shielding and background characterisation	At commissioning.
Crosstalk	At commissioning.
Decay correction	At commissioning.
Count-rate performance	At commissioning.
Sample volume effects	Perform at commissioning for each isotope and type of vial/ sample holder to be used. Repeat before new vials are used.
Database management	Quarterly/annually depending on use

instruments can be programmed to automatically check for contamination by measuring an empty sample tube prior to each batch of samples and comparing this with baseline data accumulated previously. A warning can then be issued, alerting the user to the need for instrument maintenance, to prevent incorrect background subtraction and other interference with sample counts. Where this function is not available, the background should be measured prior to and after each counting session using the same setup as the baseline measurement in order to check for radioactive contamination in the detector wells or other external sources of radioactivity. The counting time should be long enough to collect sufficient counts to minimise statistical errors. This should be in the region of 10 min unless otherwise specified by the manufacturer.

If the well(s) are contaminated they can either be left to decay (if a short half-life isotope has been used), or they should be carefully decontaminated according to the manufacturer's instructions. The background should be re-checked after decontamination to ensure it has returned to expected levels. Any increase in the background that cannot be attributed to contamination should be investigated, as it may indicate an issue with the detector or electronics.

It should be noted that sample holders can also become contaminated and it is recommended that a dedicated sample holder that is not used for transporting radioactive samples should be reserved in order to perform background checks.

4.6.4 Sensitivity

Sensitivity is one of the most important performance factors in a gamma counter and a decrease in the absolute sensitivity is an indicator of detector degradation. The sensitivity is dependent on detector characteristics, the source geometry, and the isotope measured. As such, the detector sensitivity should be measured for each radionuclide and energy window to be used. Baseline sensitivity measures of the counts per minute (CPM) per kBq should be performed at commissioning. The sensitivity measurements should then be repeated annually and after any repair, using the same energy window and geometry for comparison to the baseline values. The sensitivity (S) can be calculated as:

$$S = \frac{C - B}{A\mathrm{e}^{-\lambda \Delta t}},$$

where C is the gross sample count rate, B is the background count rate, A is the measured activity, λ is the decay constant for the isotope and Δt is the time between the activity measurement and the start of counting.

4.6.5 Constancy of sensitivity and long-term stability

The long-term stability of the instrument is particularly important if results are to be compared in longitudinal studies or to a reference standard that is not measured in the same counting session. After installation or major upgrades, measurements should be made of a long-lived radioactive source of similar energy to the samples to be counted (e.g. ^{57}Co, ^{68}Ge, ^{129}I, or ^{137}Cs). If a wide range of isotopes are routinely measured, several long-lived sources with energies spanning the clinical range to be measured should be counted. Measurements should be repeated over the course of a few days or weeks to establish the expected variation and tolerances for daily constancy measurements, as determined from the 95% confidence intervals. Before each counting session, the same long-lived radioactive source(s) should be measured using the same geometry and energy window settings as those used for previous measurements to check that the count rate is within these tolerance levels (after accounting for decay). These daily constancy of sensitivity measurements should be reviewed on a quarterly basis to look for any longer-term trends. Additional constancy measurements should be made prior to and immediately after the normalisation/re-calibration of the detectors to ensure that there are no significant jumps (>5%) in performance.

It should be noted that in addition to the photomultiplier tube, the scintillator crystal performance will be dependent on the temperature. Most commercial detectors intended to be used in a normal laboratory environment operate consistently over a wide range of temperatures, but the rate of temperature change should be minimised. Based on the temperature coefficient of light yield for NaI(Tl) of –0.3% $°C^{-1}$, the change in response to temperature is typically small. If there is a concern that the temperature variation in the laboratory is sufficient to result in significant changes in response over time, the use of a dynamic counting window can compensate for this, although caution should be used in applying this routinely (see section 4.4.3). A rapid change in temperature, however, is a greater cause for concern, as it can cause the crystal to crack due to rapid expansion and contraction. As a guide, the recommendation for NaI(Tl) is that the temperature change should not exceed 13°C per hour; this may vary for other scintillation crystals and users should refer to the manufacturer's specifications (Hibbard 1975).

4.6.6 Energy resolution and photopeak channels

The energy resolution (full width at half maximum of the photopeak) and the peak channel for the photopeak should be measured using a reference source, e.g. ^{57}Co, ^{68}Ge, ^{129}I, or ^{137}Cs. This can be performed using the same long-lived radioactive source(s) as that used for constancy measurements. Drift in the peak channel(s) indicates that normalisation should be performed to recalibrate the detectors, as outlined in section 4.6.7. Degradation of the crystal can manifest in poorer energy resolution in the long term. Many scintillation crystals used for gamma counting are hygroscopic, meaning that they are easily damaged when exposed to moisture in the air. The crystal should be hermetically sealed to prevent exposure to the air, but the seal can become compromised due to age, exposure to excessive humidity/condensation, or disturbance.

4.6.7 Normalisation

In multi-detector systems, normalisation is performed to adjust for variations in gain between detectors and achieve consistent counting efficiencies across all detectors in the sample counter. Normalisation should be performed for all isotope energies to be used. For isotopes with short half-lives, long-lived sources can be used for normalisation. For PET isotopes, a ^{68}Ge source can be purchased for normalisation.

If performing cross-calibration with other equipment, such as a PET scanner, the sample counter normalisation should be scheduled to coincide with the scanner QC.

4.6.8 Cross-calibration

In PET, blood sample counting is used in studies in which absolute quantification is required. In this case, counts from the sample counter need to be related back to the injected activity from the radionuclide calibrator and the PET scanner. As part of the routine quality control for a PET scanner, a cross-calibration factor is determined to convert the counts measured in the reconstructed PET images into an activity concentration (Bq mL^{-1}). The cross-calibration factor is measured by acquiring a PET scan of a water-filled uniform cylinder containing a known ^{18}F activity concentration. To further determine the cross-calibration factor for the sample counter, 10 aliquots should be taken from the phantom and counted in the sample counter. The activity concentration (Bq mL^{-1}) measured in the PET image can then be directly related to the CPM measured in the sample counter. The cross-calibration factor should be checked after the sample counter and the PET scanner have been normalised, which is usually performed quarterly.

4.6.9 Repeatability

Repeatability measures the test–retest reliability of the instrument for the same sample under the same conditions. A single sample should be measured using the intended clinical protocol and this same sample measured at least 20 times in succession. The repeatability is reported as the standard deviation or coefficient of variation of the measurements. To avoid issues with decay, a long-lived source can be used for this test.

In addition, a chi-squared (χ^2) goodness of fit test can be performed to check for instabilities in the instrument. The null hypothesis is that the observed variation in the measurements is consistent with those expected for a Poisson distribution. The χ^2 test returns a *p*-value between zero and one that indicates the strength of the evidence supporting the hypothesis. If the *p*-value is very small ($\leqslant 0.05$) then the probability that the random variations in the measurements come from a Poisson distribution is very low and the null hypothesis is rejected. In this case there are other sources of random variation present in the measurements.

4.6.10 Shielding and background characterisation

The purpose of this test is to investigate the effectiveness of the sample counter's shielding. The counter contains a certain amount of internal shielding, which should prevent significant penetration of radiation from external sources. Ideally, the counter should be located in a dedicated room with low background activity, away from potential external radiation sources. Additional shielding may be required in the doors or walls of the room, or around the counter, if it is sited in a storage area containing radioactive samples or waste, in order to prevent unexpected results. A radioactive source that has the total activity level expected within the counter room should be placed at strategic locations around the room and the background count repeated. This can be used to emulate waste or sample storage and determine the upper levels of radioactivity that can be processed or whether there are specific areas where radioactive sources should not be stored while counting samples.

4.6.11 Crosstalk

The crosstalk from samples in adjacent detectors and from those on the conveyor should be checked and characterised. High-activity samples (such as blood and plasma) should not be counted in the same rack as low-activity samples (such as metabolites). This is particularly important for high-energy gamma emitters. In addition, high-activity samples should not be stored next to the counter during counting.

4.6.12 Count-rate performance (linearity)

This test aims to evaluate the count-rate performance across a range of activities and to determine the upper limit of activities that can be counted before dead-time effects result in significant errors. A sample is repeatedly counted as it decays over the range of activities to be encountered. The measured count rate should be plotted as a function of activity concentration. The expected count rate is determined by extrapolating the linear least-squares fit from the lower activities (for which the dead time is assumed to be negligible) to the higher activities. The error in the count rate is determined from the difference between the measured and expected count rates (figure 4.2). If the sample counter uses a dead-time correction, this should be applied to the data to test the accuracy of the correction. Note that if ^{99m}Tc is used, discrepancies may be observed at low count rates due to the presence of ^{99}Mo.

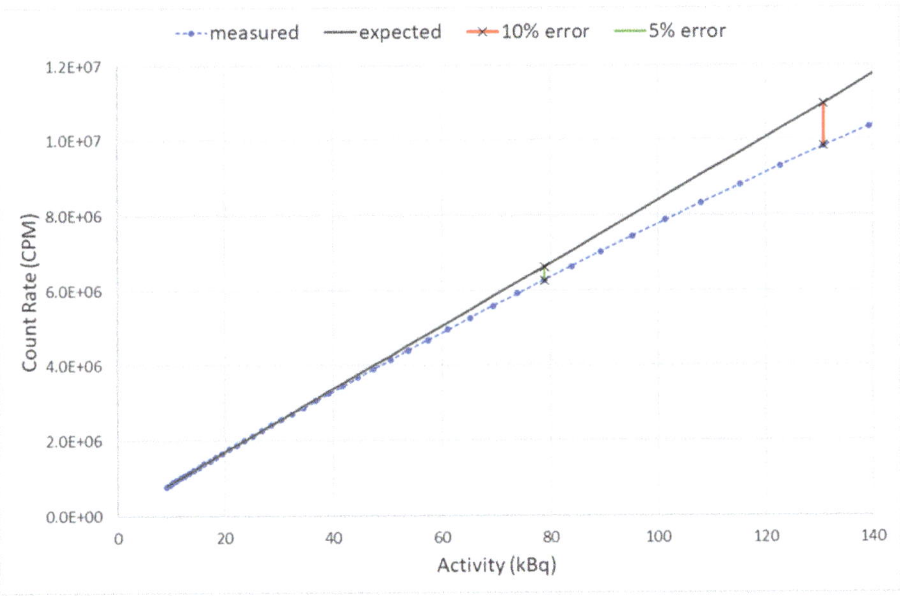

Figure 4.2. Count rate as a function of activity for ^{18}F in 1 ml using an NaI(Tl) well-type detector. At higher levels of radioactivity in the sample, dead-time effects cause the measured count rate to deviate from the expected count rate.

It should be noted that scintillation crystals, particularly NaI(Tl) and CsI(Tl), are susceptible to radiation damage if exposed to high levels of radiation. This will result in a decrease in the height of the photopeak and a decrease in the energy resolution. The likely linear range of the counter will be around 100–200 kBq and the radioactivity of clinical samples is much lower than this; therefore, the initial radioactivity used for the count-rate test should not exceed the maximum count rate quoted by the manufacturer at the start of measurement.

4.6.13 Sample volume effects

The efficiency of gamma counters depends on the geometry and positioning of the sample. In through-hole detectors, samples can be centred and so variation with sample volume is not significant below a certain volume. In well-type detectors, the fraction of the gamma rays escaping from the top of the well increases as the sample volume increases (figure 4.3). Therefore, when counting matching samples, the sample volumes and vials should be kept identical to avoid errors due to sample volume effects, particularly in well-type detectors. By assessing the sample volume effects for a specific container, the volume can be selected to provide a good balance between efficiency and volume errors due to pipetting small volumes. A more detailed discussion of the considerations for sample volume selection is provided in section 10.8.

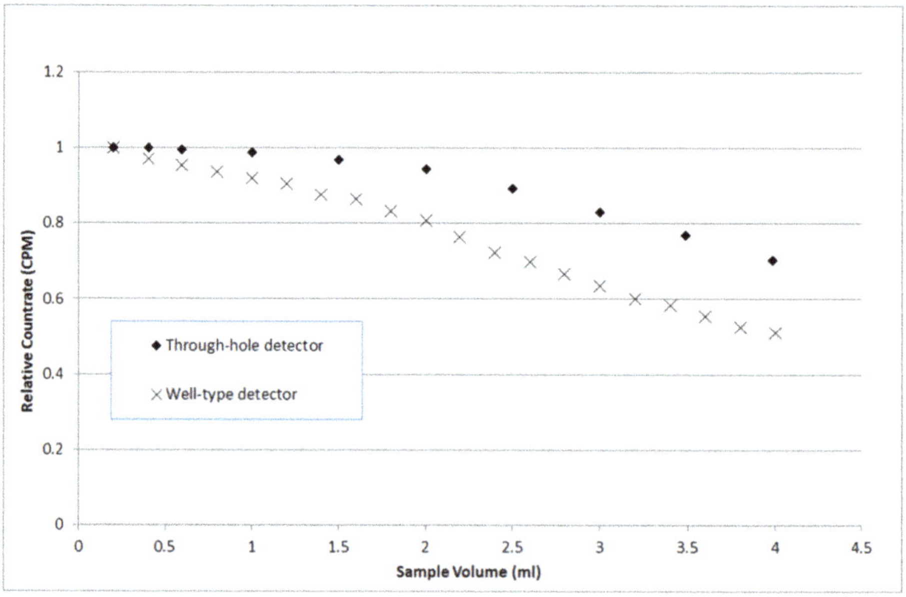

Figure 4.3. The relative count rate measured for a sample of ^{18}F with constant activity and increasing volume (counting window 400–600 keV). As the volume in the sample is increased, the relative count rate for the well-type detector decreases, as a greater fraction of the gamma rays escape from the top of the well. In the through-hole detector, samples can be centred using an elevator to reduce the fraction of gamma rays escaping and so less variation is seen for the smaller volumes.

The change in relative count rate with sample volume also depends on the isotope and energy window used and so should be tested with the specific containers used to determine the optimal volume for the application. This combination of volume, container, and window settings should be maintained to ensure consistent counts. An example of this would be the use of positron emitters or other isotopes with summation peaks; if a narrow energy window around the main photopeak is used, this can reduce sample volume effects, but would result in a loss in overall sensitivity compared to using a wider window that encompasses the summation peak (Lodge *et al* 2015).

The impact of sample volume should be tested by first counting a small volume (e.g. 0.2 mL) containing radioactivity within the range where dead-time effects are minimal. The sample should be re-counted after progressively diluting it with water (up to 4.0 mL) whilst keeping the total activity the same. The count rates should be corrected for any decay relative to the first sample.

Sample volume effects are dependent on the energy and type of emission; low-energy sources such as ^{125}I (27–35 keV) also suffer from absorption within the sample and the walls of the vial. Therefore, sample volume effects should be investigated for all vials to be used and across the range of isotopes to be counted. If the sample vials are changed (size, shape, or material) the sample volume effects should be retested for the new vials.

A worked example of evaluating a change in counter efficiency with sample volume for ^{99m}Tc is included in section 10.8.

4.6.14 Database management

Some sample counters use a local database; if many samples are counted, this may fill up quickly. Regular database reviews should be performed and older results should be deleted or archived in a secure location according to local data retention policies. The ability to connect the counter to a local area network would provide a simple and secure way to export data for long-term storage.

4.6.15 Service contracts

Routine service dates should be scheduled and an accurate description of any problems that have occurred should be presented to the service engineer. In addition, enquire on a yearly basis whether the manufacturer has developed any improvements or modifications for this particular model that should be considered.

Preventative maintenance visits (annual) should include:

1. PC and software checks, including database maintenance and backup of protocols/settings.
2. Cleaning and checks of mechanical parts (motors, fans, conveyor, etc).
3. Inspection of electronic components.
4. Full set of calibrations and review of software tolerances.

As part of the equipment handover, the routine quality control checks (background, energy resolution, and constancy) should be performed after the service to ensure consistent performance.

References

Hibbard W M 1975 Effects of temperature changes on NaI crystals *J. Nucl. Med. Technol.* **3** 168–9

HIDEX Automatic Gamma Counter User Guide, Software Version 1.2.16.0 2017

Lodge M A, Holt D P, Kinahan P E, Wong D F and Wahl R L 2015 Performance assessment of a NaI (Tl) gamma counter for PET applications with methods for improved quantitative accuracy and greater standardization *EJNMMI Phys.* **2** 11

NHS 2010 NHS terms and conditions: procuring goods and services https://www.gov.uk/government/publications/nhs-standard-terms-and-conditions-of-contract-for-the-purchase-of-goods-and-supply-of-services

PerkinElmer 2002 PerkinElmer Wallac 1470 Wizard Gamma Counter Instrument Manual

Chapter 5

Intraoperative gamma probes

Anne-Marie Stapleton and Fergus McKiddie

5.1 Introduction to gamma probe instrumentation

Gamma probe systems are based around a small detection probe which is sensitive to gamma photons, and which shows the user either the counts detected or the subsequent count rate in a given energy window. The electrical signal resulting from a detection event is then transmitted either via Bluetooth or a cable to a base unit which counts these signals, and the user display shows either the count rate or total counts in a given time period. In some systems, the counts recorded may be processed within the handheld probe itself and displayed directly on a screen on the probe. As well as displaying the total integrated counts or count rate observed by the probe, these probes also have a variable audible signal to indicate the instantaneous count rate.

5.2 Clinical applications of gamma probes

Gamma probes are typically used during surgery to locate discrete areas of radioactivity *in vivo*. The patient is injected with a radiopharmaceutical which localises in the area of interest. The probe is then used during surgery to establish where the detected counts are maximised and therefore indicate where the radioactivity has localised.

A common use of gamma probes is in the detection and localisation of sentinel nodes during surgery, in order to enable the removal of the first lymph node that a known cancerous tumour drains to. This node may then be tested to establish histologically whether the cancer has spread into the lymphatic system. If the node tests positive for cancer, this may result in the removal of additional lymph nodes, whereas if the sentinel node does not demonstrate the spread of the cancer to the lymphatic system, the remaining healthy lymph nodes may be spared. Sentinel node localisation occurs for a range of malignancies including breast, vulvar, and penile

doi:10.1088/978-0-7503-3895-0ch5

cancer as well as malignant melanoma (Schneebaum *et al* 1999). Patients are often given their radioactive injection prior to surgery and have been imaged using a gamma camera to establish the initial lymphatic drainage, to assist the surgeon in the location of the lymph node(s) of interest.

Gamma probe systems may also be applied in the detection and location of parathyroid glands to facilitate a successful minimally invasive radioguided parathyroidectomy. Additionally, they may be used with PET tracers such as F-18-FDG for FDG-avid tumour localisation (Gulec *et al* 2016).

For a more complete description of a range of gamma probe applications, see Povoski *et al* (2009).

5.3 Gamma probe types

5.3.1 Detector types

Gamma probe systems detect gamma rays using a small sensitive detector at the end of a probe. The detectors may be small inorganic scintillator crystals, such as thallium-doped sodium iodide NaI(Tl) or thallium-doped caesium iodide CsI(Tl). These produce light that is detected by a PMT and converted into an electrical signal as described in chapter 2. Alternatively, the detector in the probe may be semiconductor based, for example using cadmium zinc telluride (CZT). Semiconductor probes tend to have a smaller diameter and are often sensitive to a narrower energy range of emitted gammas compared to inorganic crystal-based detectors, allowing for better scatter rejection, but have a lower sensitivity overall, especially for medium- and high-energy gamma radiation (Povoski *et al* 2009).

5.3.2 Probe unit types

The most common types of gamma probe system consist of a reusable handheld probe which is connected to a remote base unit. The base unit tends to be plugged into the mains electricity to supply continuous power to the system, although fully battery-powered systems exist. Some base units are capable of being connected to multiple probes simultaneously and selecting a probe for use, allowing probes with different characteristics in terms of size, shape, resolution, and sensitivity (amongst other things) to be used during the same surgery. Others only have one connection available between the probe and the base unit, so whilst probes can be changed at the base unit, this would not tend to happen during a given surgery. Reusable probes are used clinically with disposable sterile sheaths to allow for effective cleaning and decontamination between patients.

5.3.3 Connection between the probe and base unit

In systems that have a probe with a wired connection to the base unit, the probe receives power from the mains. This physical connection between the two minimises the risk of the probe accidentally being disposed of with other disposable surgical equipment.

Other systems have a Bluetooth connection between the probe and base unit, allowing for less constrained probe movement during surgery, and reducing the problems associated with having trailing cables in the area. However, the lack of a cable increases the risk of the probe being dropped and damaged, or being inadvertently disposed of with the other consumables following surgery. Occasionally, these systems may suffer from communication interference issues due to the presence of other electrical equipment or mobile phones. Bluetooth probes use semiconductor detectors and are battery powered. Due to the power demands of the detectors, the battery levels must always be checked prior to commencing surgery.

Other self-contained probe systems exist, in which the handheld probe itself contains all of the necessary counting circuitry and provides a display of the total counts in the probe handle. In this case, the probe is again battery powered, and the battery level requires checking prior to clinical use.

5.3.4 Collimators

Probes usually have removable collimators, which may be made of lead or tungsten. Clinically, it is recommended that probes are always used with an appropriate collimator, depending on the application in question. Collimators improve spatial and angular resolution and improve scatter rejection, leading to an improved ability of the probe to accurately localise the area of interest. This reduces the apparent sensitivity of the probe, but may increase confidence that a maximum in the detected counts is indicative that a region of increased activity has been found.

5.3.5 Disposable gamma probe systems

Recent advances in gamma probe systems have resulted in the development of single-use disposable gamma probes. These are currently available in two types: a more traditional handheld type (Hologic Website 2021) and a smaller tethered probe type which is suitable for robotic or manual laparoscopic surgery, as well as for open procedures (Sensei Surgical Website 2021). Versions of such probes available at the time of writing include a reusable base unit and sterile single-use probes. These sterile probes have in-built collimation and shielding. The probes can either connect to the base unit via a Bluetooth connection, in which case the probe has an in-built battery, or via a cable, which may deliver power from the base unit to the probe.

The advantage of disposable probes is that they are fully sterile for surgery, thereby reducing the risk of cross-contamination and surgical site infections. However, single-use probes only allow a limited time for commissioning and testing prior to clinical use, which must be performed in a sterile field. Additionally, for Bluetooth-connected probes, battery life can further limit the duration for which the probe can be used; current systems offer approximately 1–2 h. Given that these probes are disposable, along with the time and potential complexity of commissioning each probe in a sterile field, the overall cost must be considered prior to the purchase of these systems. Additionally, it would not be advisable for a single site to use a combination of disposable and reusable probes for the same procedures within the same setting, as there could be an increased risk of the reusable probes accidentally being disposed of by force of habit.

5.4 Counting options

In comparison with a well-type gamma counter, gamma probes are significantly less sensitive in detecting gamma photons as a result of their smaller detector size and reduced geometric efficiency between the source and the detector. However, they are well suited to their role in surgery, as they are relatively small, light, manoeuvrable, easy to clean, and have an audible signal proportional to the detection count rate, allowing the user to easily monitor the gamma-ray detected count rate without having to look at the display screen.

5.4.1 Squelch

In a gamma probe, squelch effectively removes a set number of background counts from those detected. The user finds an area of background radiation and if at that point they activate the squelch function, this background count rate is then removed from the subsequent count rates detected. As an example, if the probe is measuring a background count rate of 50 counts per second (cps) and squelch is then enabled, a source that the probe would have measured as 150 cps actually records (150 cps – 50 cps) = 100 cps.

5.4.2 Energy window

Most systems have a number of manufacturer-defined selectable energy windows available for the user, depending on the possible applications of the probe system. Some systems allow for additional user-defined energy windows to be created. Having a probe set up with a narrower energy window has the benefit that it will detect fewer counts due to scattered and background radiation compared to the same probe with a wider energy window. However, this may come at the expense of probe sensitivity to true emissions, depending on the energy resolution of the probe and the actual energy window width.

5.4.3 Counting time

Gamma probe systems have two ways in which gamma-ray detections are displayed: either as an instantaneous count rate, or as the total integrated count over a set time period. A typical available range in counting time is between 1 and 60 s, with a time of ~10 s often used as a standard integration time. The integration time can usually be adjusted to accommodate the clinical or testing situation in which the probe is used.

5.5 Specification and purchase of gamma probes

With the increasing prevalence of sentinel lymph node examinations using different radionuclides and for varied cancer types, it becomes ever more important that the intraoperative gamma probes used are appropriate for the task and are properly maintained.

Guidelines and procurement questionnaires are available (BNMS 2004) to assist with the selection and evaluation of suitable devices. The following are recommended for consideration when a gamma probe system is to be purchased:

- probe types required versus those available, including the probe shapes, sizes, and sensitivities, available detectors, and connection method to base unit (if relevant)
- preset energy windows required versus those available and the possibility of creating additional user-defined energy windows if required
- whether probe energy calibration (described in section 5.5.1) is required as part of the daily test—this has the potential to increase the variance in daily test results
- whether the base unit can connect to more than one probe during a single surgery, and the likelihood of whether this is useful or would be used clinically
- collimator options available
- ease of probe cleaning and decontamination method; as both radioactive and biological contaminations may occur, it is advisable to liaise with the local infection control team to determine the most appropriate decontamination method
- type of clinical use, for example, laparoscopic or open surgery
- ease of clinical use, given the desired application
- expected frequency of clinical use—this may be of particular relevance in the consideration of whether to procure a system with a disposable probe
- ease of readout of display—some screens may have high reflectivity, which can cause a glare under the bright lights present in theatres, rendering the readout difficult to see
- ease of testing, including commissioning
- cost of probe(s) and base unit
- cost of radioactive sources required for quality assurance
- cost of servicing/repair
- data management of recorded counts, i.e. must counts be recorded from the screen at the time of acquisition, or are they recallable at the end of the session?
- supplier training provision and availability
- amount, frequency, and detail of further training that may be required for theatre staff to support testing and clinical use
- support available from the manufacturer following purchase and warranty details of the probe

5.6 Quality assurance

All probes purchased should be properly tested at commissioning prior to clinical use to establish baseline values of the parameters of interest under the oversight of an

Table 5.1. Recommended quality control tests and frequencies for gamma probes.

Test	Suggested frequency
Cleaning and decontamination	Daily/weekly depending on use and between patients
Power check and visual inspection	Prior to each session
Background checks	Baseline measured at commissioning; prior to each session
Constancy of sensitivity and long-term stability	Tolerances set at commissioning or after major upgrade; constancy of sensitivity measured prior to counting session and long-term stability reviewed quarterly
Short-term stability	Measured at commissioning, quarterly, and following repairs
Energy window check	Measured at commissioning, quarterly, and following repairs
Sensitivity in air	Baseline measured at commissioning, annually, and following repairs
Count-rate performance (linearity)	At commissioning/post repair if deemed necessary
Sensitivity in scatter	At commissioning (see NEMA 2004)
Shielding and background characterisation	At commissioning (see NEMA 2004)

MPE. The National Electrical Manufacturer's Association (NEMA) provides detailed guidelines for appropriate testing to be conducted as part of the thorough acceptance testing of gamma probes (NEMA 2004). The measured results should be compared to the manufacturer's specification or type test data, where available. The performance of probes often varies, and it is important to determine the baseline performance at the time of commissioning using repeated measurements to define variability. These baseline measurements will then determine the tolerance levels for system performance for daily QC, taking into account differences in specification between different probe types and manufacturers.

Regular quality control tests for gamma probes are essential to ensure appropriate function during surgery. Gamma probes are typically relatively fragile compared to other counting systems, and therefore may be expected to require repair during their working lifetime. Faults may develop in the detector itself, such as a crystal that is cracked as a result of physical trauma to the probe, or in the wiring and connectors linking the probe to the base unit, amongst other things. Testing following repair benefits from having baseline values which were recorded at acceptance for comparison, in particular, the sensitivity and spatial resolution may be of particular interest. Published guidance for the quality control of gamma probes is provided by both the British and European Nuclear Medicine Associations (BNMS 2004, Busemann Sokole *et al* 2010). The remainder of this chapter outlines essential daily and periodic quality control procedures for gamma probe systems. It is recommended that the tests given are performed at the frequencies given in table 5.1.

5.6.1 Daily quality control

The daily tests should be carried out each time the probe is to be used in the theatre environment, although this may be less frequently than daily in practice, depending on the clinical need. Ideally, the probe should be switched on and allowed to acclimatise to ambient conditions for around 15 min or more prior to testing or use.

Some systems require calibration on each day of use to ensure that the isotope energy detected is correctly assigned, using a known long-lived radioactive check source as part of a manufacturer-defined in-built system test. Other systems do not require this to be done, and in either case, a daily test is recommended as described in the checks below.

5.6.1.1 Power

The cable(s) and plugs or connectors of mains-powered systems should be checked for visual signs of damage. Some systems indicate voltage problems on the display screen and prevent counts from being acquired or tests from being performed. In this case, internal electronics or cable faults may be indicated.

Systems powered by rechargeable batteries or those with separate probes, i.e. Bluetooth-connected systems, should be fully charged on first use to ensure optimal battery utilisation, then recharged before each surgical use, always as per the manufacturer's guidance. The status of the battery charge should be visually checked before each surgical use. For systems with permanent non-rechargeable batteries, the status of the battery charge should again be visually checked before each surgical use to ascertain the remaining battery life. As the charge drops to a predetermined level, say 20% of the maximum, contingency plans should be put in place to return the system to the manufacturer for battery replacement. This obviously requires the possession of, or access to, a backup gamma probe system to ensure continuation of the surgical service. This contingency may be considered as part of system purchase or as an ongoing contract with the manufacturer.

5.6.1.2 Visual inspection

The casing and outer surfaces of the probe should be checked for cracks or chips which may allow moisture to enter or compromise the integrity of the sterile surgical sheaths. This is particularly important around the probe tip, where external damage may correlate with internal damage to the crystal or semiconductor detector. For systems which have a base unit, this should also be inspected for damage and the visual and audible display systems checked for correct operation. All additional cabling and connectors should also be checked for damage to the insulation, broken wiring, or crush damage, to ensure correct operation and that electrical safety is not compromised.

5.6.1.3 Background check

Prior to use, a background check should be performed in which an integrated count is taken using the clinical energy window and settings, in the absence of any radioactive sources or patients that have been injected with radiopharmaceuticals. The total counts due to background should be very low and stable. Higher counts may indicate that the probe is contaminated with radioactivity or a radioactive source may be in the near vicinity of the probe. Other problems can be detected by this check including, but not limited to, spurious electrical noise, problems with the cable or connectors (if relevant), or interference affecting the Bluetooth connection between the base unit and probe (where relevant). All of these situations warrant further investigation prior to clinical use.

5.6.1.4 Constancy of sensitivity and long-term stability

The measurement of probe sensitivity is the most important check made during the daily test. Issues with equipment sensitivity could indicate faults in a number of subsystems, such as crystal or detector damage, change in electrical gain, energy window drift, or an electronics fault. The test is intended to demonstrate that the sensitivity of the probe is reproducible over time if all equipment settings are kept constant. This test can therefore also achieve the outcomes covered by other measures mentioned in some of the guidelines, such as constancy (Busemann Sokole et al 2010) and energy window drift (BNMS 2004). Sensitivity is expressed in counts per second per unit activity (e.g. cps MBq^{-1}).

Measuring the constancy of sensitivity is best achieved by measuring a long-lived sealed source in a reproducible geometry. Systems optimised for the detection of PET emitters may use a positron-emitting ^{22}Na check source as a long-lived sealed source for constancy testing (C-Trak manual). ^{57}Co is frequently used for probes optimised for detecting ^{99m}Tc and other relatively low-energy gamma emitters. ^{57}Co has a relatively long physical half-life (270 days) and gamma-energy emission at 122 keV. This is sufficiently close to the photopeak energy of ^{99m}Tc at $E = 141$ keV that the manufacturer preset clinical energy window for ^{99m}Tc will often overlap with the ^{57}Co photopeak, and a detectable count rate will be obtained with most commercially available systems. This data could also be recorded on a Shewhart chart (section 3.3) to monitor device stability.

That said, some systems exist in which sealed-source ^{57}Co gamma emissions may be unacceptably rejected by a relatively narrow preset ^{99m}Tc clinical energy window. Here, the ^{57}Co energy peak is at an energy either partially or completely outside the predefined clinical energy window. This potentially increases the complexity of QC testing, as it may require a different source to be used or the energy window to be changed for the purpose of QC, which poses a clinical risk that the probe will not be returned to the correct energy window for clinical use. In such a case, a user-defined energy window may be created to allow the detection of both the ^{99m}Tc and ^{57}Co photopeaks and therefore used for clinical as well as QC purposes. This change should enable effective determination of the constancy of sensitivity and reduce likely errors in the sensitivity value measured using ^{57}Co. As the new ^{99m}Tc energy window is used throughout, there is no risk that the probe energy window will be left on the ^{57}Co setting for surgery after the daily constancy check. Following such an adjustment to system energy windows, the gamma probe should be carefully tested

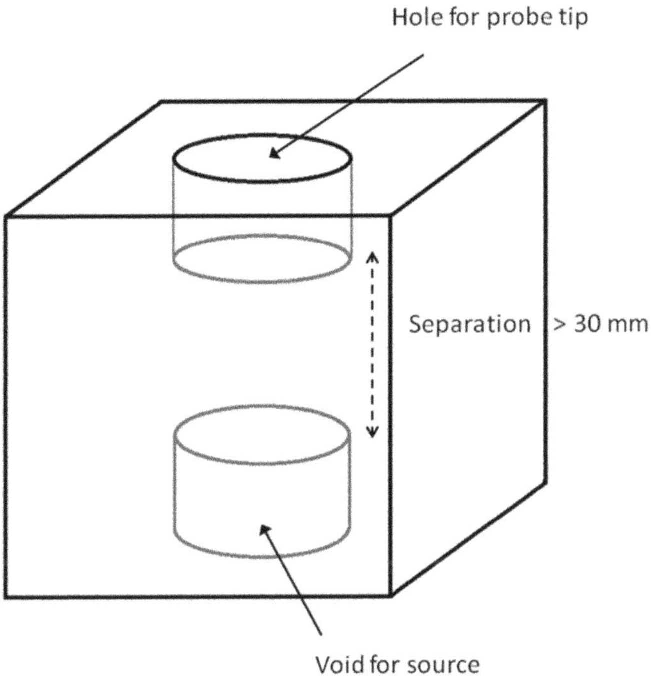

Figure 5.1. Schematic of a possible test block design for gamma probe quality control

to ensure that its other detection properties, such as its spatial resolution, have not been unacceptably changed. Typically, a tolerance of ±10% or two standard deviations (SD) from the baseline is used for assessing the constancy of sensitivity. Some systems recalibrate the energy peak at the time of testing, which can impact the perceived constancy of sensitivity.

^{57}Co sealed sources, often in the form of spot markers and with activities generally between 1 and 3.7 MBq at the beginning of their lifespan, are readily available in most Nuclear Medicine departments and can otherwise be purchased for a few hundred pounds. The source should be positioned at a fixed distance from the tip of the probe, generally approximately 3 cm away, to give reproducible results. Although this may be done in air, it is best done in the presence of a scatter material to accurately reflect the clinical situation. To achieve this, a simple Perspex or polycarbonate test block can be manufactured with apertures for the probe tip and the source (see figure 5.1). Many commercial gamma probe manufacturers provide a spot source holder with the probe when it is purchased to enable reproducible sensitivity measurements. These give a fixed geometry between the probe tip and source, which may be less than 3 cm. In either case, when the count rates measured are high, the user should be mindful of the potential for dead-time effects (especially when counting is performed in air) and if they are significant, consider whether it is either necessary to increase the distance between the source and the probe, or to use a lower-activity source. If this is not possible, and the dead time is significant and unavoidable, the constancy of sensitivity test limits will need to be reset periodically (typically quarterly), as the dead time reduces and therefore the apparent gamma probe sensitivity improves. As sources decay to give lower count rates, consideration may be given to using smaller fixed probe-to-source distances in order to ensure that adequate counts are still acquired during this test and to prolong the useful life of the source.

Another potential source of error in this test can arise if it is performed with the source just in front of a highly scattering material, as the measured count rates may appear higher than expected.

If the routine testing is to be carried out outside the Nuclear Medicine department, for example, within the surgical department, then the issue of sealed source security must be considered. A lockable source store must be found and designated as such and a logbook or other record of access must be established. Staff will also require adequate training, and a simple method of recording the test results should be put in place, along with a procedure to be followed if the equipment fails. Arrangements for leak testing the sealed sources are required, for example, the physics team can perform leak testing during site visits and take the wipes to their main hospital for counting.

A fixed period of counting to measure a minimum of 1000 counts (to give an acceptable inherent statistical variation) should be established and either the cps or the total counts within the period should be recorded. Some systems only allow a short, fixed counting time, e.g. 10 s, in which case it may be necessary to repeat this count interval several times to collect a total of at least 1000 counts. It is generally advisable to use the same count interval as is used clinically, in order to ensure that the probe is not inadvertently left at the wrong settings after the quality control tests. If different settings are used for the counting interval, the system should be restored to the clinical settings on completion of the quality testing. Before the QA programme is rolled out, the reference value should be established by repeating the standard measurement several (e.g. 20) times or by increasing the acquired counts to at least 10 000 counts in a set time. The calculated count rate (cps) should be recorded as the reference value and decay corrected for future recordings. Measured readings should not deviate by more than 2 SD from the expected value. The measurement should be repeated if this occurs, and if the reading remains more than 2 SD from the reference value then investigative action should be taken. Faults may be indicated by either a fall in counts (a reduction in sensitivity) or a rise in counts (increased sensitivity), and all changes in sensitivity, both gain and loss, must be investigated with guidance (where required) from an MPE. A basic gamma probe troubleshooting guide is given in appendix B.

5.6.2 Periodic quality control

There are a number of tests which could be carried out on a less frequent basis for reusable probes, such as at quarterly or annual intervals, or after significant repair of a probe. An MPE should be consulted about the required testing regime for a given probe. The list below is not exhaustive, and any test used in the acceptance testing of new systems could be used to assess equipment periodically or after maintenance. Any results should be compared to the baseline values measured as part of the original gamma probe commissioning and the manufacturer-provided system specification, if available.

5.6.2.1 Repeatability

The aim is to assess the counting repeatability of the system, which indicates its short-term stability. Counts are recorded for a fixed time period (e.g. 10 s), and this is repeated a number of times ($\geqslant$20) using a long-lived check source in a fixed geometry; the chi-squared goodness-of-fit test is then used to assess the outcome (as described in section 4.6.9). The total counts collected in each counting period should be in excess of 1000. The subsequent spread of total counts should lie within the 95% confidence interval. The repeatability is reported as the standard deviation or coefficient of variation of the measurements, and the chi-squared value reported. This test should be performed quarterly or following any probe system repairs.

5.6.2.2 Sensitivity in air

The sensitivity of the probe should be assessed in a repeatable geometry using any clinically used isotope, such as ^{99m}Tc, ^{123}I, or ^{18}F and the corresponding clinical energy window(s). The activity of the source and geometry setup should be such that no dead-time effects are expected to be induced in the gamma probe (i.e. $<$1000 cps). The sensitivity may be reported in terms of counts per second per unit activity in the set geometry. Significant deviations (typically over 10% or a locally determined limit) in the measured sensitivity may indicate problems in the probe hardware or electronics. It is recommended that this test be performed annually and following any repairs which may impact system sensitivity, such as detector replacement.

5.6.2.3 Spatial resolution in air

This is a check which can be carried out with a ^{57}Co or ^{22}Na pen source if available, or a small ^{99m}Tc or ^{18}F point source. The source position is fixed and the probe is placed a given distance, say 3 cm, from the source, in accordance with the NEMA testing procedure. Counts are acquired for a fixed duration at a range of lateral distances away from the centre line of the probe axis. These can be plotted to show the spatial resolution profile and the interpolated full width at half maximum (FWHM) and full width at tenth maximum (FWTM) values can be reported and compared to the results obtained when the system was commissioned. The results obtained should typically be within 10% of those measured at commissioning.

5.6.2.4 Energy window check

Where multiple manufacturer or user windows are available, counts may be measured in each available energy window using any relevant check sources available, for example ^{57}Co or ^{22}Na, to check that the expected window records the highest counts. If when user-defined energy windows can be created, a suitable alternative is to set up and measure counts over a fixed time period in three energy windows, one centred on the expected energy peak position, a second above the peak and a third below the peak. The counts recorded in the three windows can be checked and reported to confirm whether the system is assigning the energy of the gamma photons to the central energy window as expected. This test can be performed quarterly or following repair.

5.6.2.5 Count-rate performance (activity linearity)

The aim of this check is to assess the system response to a full range of activity values and to ensure that this follows a linear distribution. The simplest way to achieve this is to start with an initial high-activity (⩾10 MBq) source of ^{99m}Tc or ^{18}F and repeat measurements in an identical geometry periodically as the source decays over a number (~10 or more) of half-lives. However, this can be time-consuming and if deemed to be impractical then a series of different activity sources, covering a sufficient activity range, can be used instead. Care should be taken to ensure that these sources have a consistent geometry to minimise the introduction of additional causes of variability. The fixed time count results should be plotted against activity and the activity linearity assessed using the correlation coefficient (with a typical tolerance level of r>0.95). As this check is, in practical terms, quite difficult to perform, it is generally only carried out during commissioning and after the probe has been repaired.

5.6.2.6 Summary of recommended quality control of gamma probes

References

BNMS 2004 *Intraoperative Gamma Probe Procurement Document (2004)—Standard Specification Questionnaire* (UK Gamma Probe Working Group) April 2004

Busemann Sokole E *et al* 2010 Routine quality control recommendations for nuclear medicine instrumentation *EJNMMI* **37** 662–71

Gulec S A, Daghighian F and Essner R 2016 PET-probe: evaluation of technical performance and clinical utility of a handheld high-energy gamma probe in oncologic surgery *Ann. Surg. Oncol.* **23** 9020–7

Hologic Website 2021 https://www.hologic.com/hologic-products/breast-health-solutions/trunode_system

NEMA 2004 Standards Publication NU 3-2004 performance measurements and quality control guidelines for non-imaging intraoperative gamma probes https://www.nema.org/standards/view/performance-measurements-and-quality-control-guidelines-for-non-imaging-intra-operative-gamma-probes)

Povoski S P *et al* 2009 A comprehensive overview of radioguided surgery using gamma detection probe technology *World J. Surg. Oncol.* **7** 11

Schneebaum S *et al* 1999 Clinical applications of gamma-detection probes—radioguided surgery *Eur. J. Nucl. Med.* **26** S26–35

Sensei Surgical Website 2021 https://senseisurgical.com/

IOP Publishing

Radioactive Sample Counting: Principles and Practice
(Second Edition)
IPEM report 85
Sofia Michopoulou

Chapter 6

Liquid scintillation counting

Anne-Marie Stapleton

6.1 Introduction

Liquid scintillation counters are predominantly used to detect alpha and beta emissions, which produce distinctly different pulse height spectra and can therefore be easily distinguished from each other. The radioactive sample is dissolved in the liquid scintillator, which consists of a mixture of several components: solvents, scintillators (also known as solutes or fluors) and additives/surfactants, to make up the liquid scintillation cocktail (Edler 2015). The original cocktails used were considered hazardous to store and use. Much effort has been invested in developing safer, more environmentally friendly scintillation cocktails with higher flash points. These are often based on long-chain aromatic derivatives with emulsifiers that help with dissolving aqueous samples.

The energy absorbed from the alpha or beta particles is converted by the scintillator into light photons which are detected by two or more adjacent PMTs. The intensity of the light produced by the scintillator is a function of the energy absorbed. The subsequent current pulse from the PMTs in the electrical circuit, corresponding to each alpha or beta particle, has a size which is approximately proportional to its energy.

The detection of gamma rays in these counters is reliant on the production of secondary electrons produced when gamma rays liberate orbital electrons, which subsequently act in the same way as beta particles in the liquid scintillation cocktail. The transfer of energy from the electron, alpha particle, or beta particle to the PMT passes through several stages, which are summarised in figure 6.1.

Up until now, pure beta-emitting radionuclides have been the main focus for clinical applications of liquid scintillation counting (Birks 1964, Horrocks 1974, Peng *et al* 1980, Ross *et al* 1991, L'Annunziata 2012). The most common of these have been ^{14}C and ^{3}H. As developments continue with radionuclide therapies using alpha emitters such as ^{211}At, ^{223}Ra, ^{225}Ac/^{213}Bi (Kozempel *et al* 2018), these nuclides amongst others may prove to be of interest for future clinical applications of liquid scintillation counting.

doi:10.1088/978-0-7503-3895-0ch6

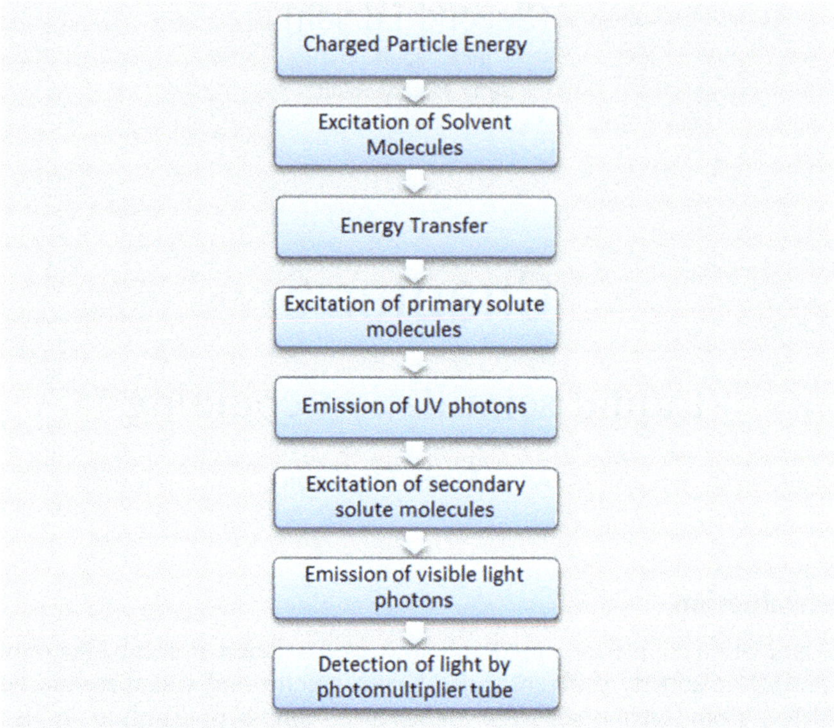

Figure 6.1. Schematic diagram of the process of energy conversion from alpha or beta particles to the detection of light by the photomultiplier tube.

6.1.1 The pulse size spectrum

The energy conversion processes in a liquid scintillation cocktail are linear, such that the pulse size(s) produced in the photomultiplier tube(s) is proportional to the energy lost in the scintillator. The pulse produced has prompt and delayed components due to de-excitation from excited singlet and triplet states, respectively. The efficiency of light output for liquid scintillators is considerably less than for sodium iodide (typically five photons per keV of energy). This limits the detectability of low-energy beta emitters such as tritium, as the pulse sizes are comparable to those produced due to thermal noise in the photomultiplier tube. Cooling the samples and counting the pulses in the two or more photomultipliers in coincidence can improve the detection of true events above the random noise.

Different pulse shapes are produced by different types of nuclear disintegration. Alpha particles are monoenergetic, and, due to their greater mass and larger charge when compared to a beta particle, do not transfer energy as efficiently to the solvent and scintillator. They produce a single pulse height, with an energy of approximately one tenth of the original alpha-decay energy (Horrocks 1974, L'Annunziata 2012). That said, the efficiency of detection of alpha events is close to 100%, even in the presence of quenching (PerkinElmer Website 2020a). The energy of beta particles

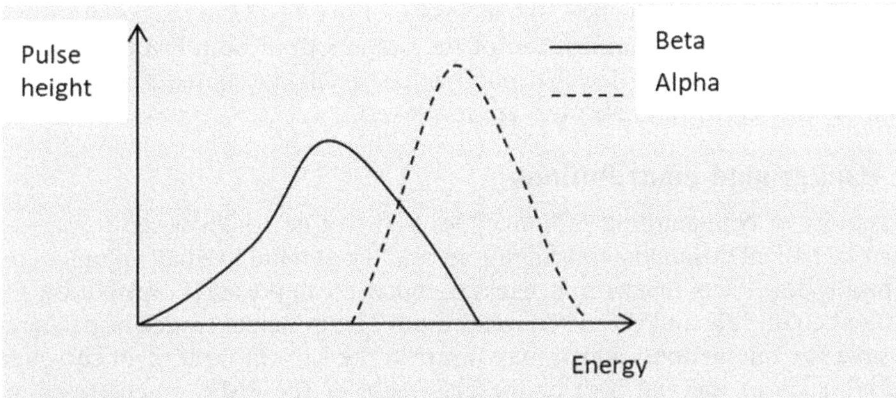

Figure 6.2. Typical alpha and beta pulse height spectrums.

emitted by a decaying nucleus has a continuous spectrum from zero up to a maximum energy, and this is reflected in the pulse height spectrum. Typical alpha and beta spectrums obtained using a liquid scintillation counter are shown in figure 6.2.

The differences in the pulse height spectra for alpha and beta emissions may be used, for example, to count the activities of alpha- and beta-emitting radionuclides in a sample containing a mixture of both (Passo and Cook 1994). The beta events are also characterised by a shorter time duration of scintillation light in the cocktail than alpha events, meaning that the different types of event can be separated by analysing the pulse decay time (PerkinElmer Website 2020a). Given that the beta pulse size is proportional to energy loss, two different beta emitters may be counted simultaneously (section 6.11).

6.1.2 Coincidence detection

Since low-energy radionuclides produce only a small number of photoelectrons at the PMT photocathode, background noise is often significant and occurs due to spontaneous thermal emission from the photocathode and phosphorescence of the scintillation solution. Coincidence detection is one of the most effective methods of reducing background noise.

In LSC systems optical reflectors are placed around the counting vial and reflect the light into two opposing PMTs. Pulses from each tube pass via separate preamplifiers to a coincidence unit. Pulses occurring within a predefined time (typically 0.2 μs) are considered to originate from the same event, in which case, a gate allows the summed signal through. If the time limit is exceeded, the pulses are rejected. The use of coincidence circuitry reduces background noise by a factor of 10^4. However, some random noise coincidences (R_C) still occur at a rate given by:

$$R_C = 2\tau R_n^2,$$

where τ is the resolving time of the coincidence circuit and R_n is the noise pulse rate for each PMT (assumed to be equal).

In addition to noise reduction, the inclusion of two PMTs in the counting system has a further advantage. Summation of the outputs from both PMTs results in an increase in the number of detected photons per event. In consequence, the energy resolution and signal-to-noise ratio are improved.

6.2 Background contributions

The activity of beta-emitting radionuclides that can be administered to patients is limited by patient dosimetry considerations and the amount in small volume samples is typically low. This means that background is an important contribution to the measured count rate and should be minimised. The principal source of background is cosmic ray interactions, which may occur in the solvent itself or in surrounding material, such as the vial wall or the glass case of the PMT. Interactions in the surroundings are detected via the emission of secondary electrons or Cerenkov radiation (section 6.11).

Natural radioactivity represents a smaller but important component of background. Thin-walled plastic vials are preferable to glass in this respect, as they contain smaller quantities of radioactive potassium (^{40}K), but they can only be used for cocktails that do not react with the plastic. Instrument noise and crosstalk between the PMTs can result in added signal background. (Passo and Cook 1994).

6.3 Energy losses in liquid scintillation

6.3.1 Quenching

The efficiency of energy transfer in the solvent–scintillator system is affected by quenching, i.e. any mechanism that reduces the energy output from the sample being detected in the PMTs. In order to reduce the effect of noise in the pulse height spectrum, an energy window is used, which is defined by lower and upper energy discriminators. As quenching reduces the light output, it shifts the pulse height spectrum downwards (figure 6.3), which may reduce the number of scintillation photons detected above the lower-energy threshold that has been set at the upper end of the noise spectrum. This effect is more marked for low-energy emitters. Therefore, counting efficiency will vary with the nature of the sample, the scintillator used, and the method of preparation of the sample. It is essential to monitor the counting efficiency for each sample if comparisons with standards or other samples are to be meaningful. This is done by measuring the amount of quenching taking place, which enables the detected count rate to be related to the disintegration rate in the sample and hence to sample activity.

There are four principal types of quenching:

1. Physical quenching resulting from the physical separation of the radionuclide from the scintillator (PerkinElmer Website 2020b). The solution here is to ensure that the solution is fully homogenised;
2. Chemical quenching (sometimes called impurity quenching) which is caused by substances that compete with the primary scintillator for absorption of energy from the solvent but are not scintillators. Dissolved oxygen is a common example of a substance that causes this type of quenching;

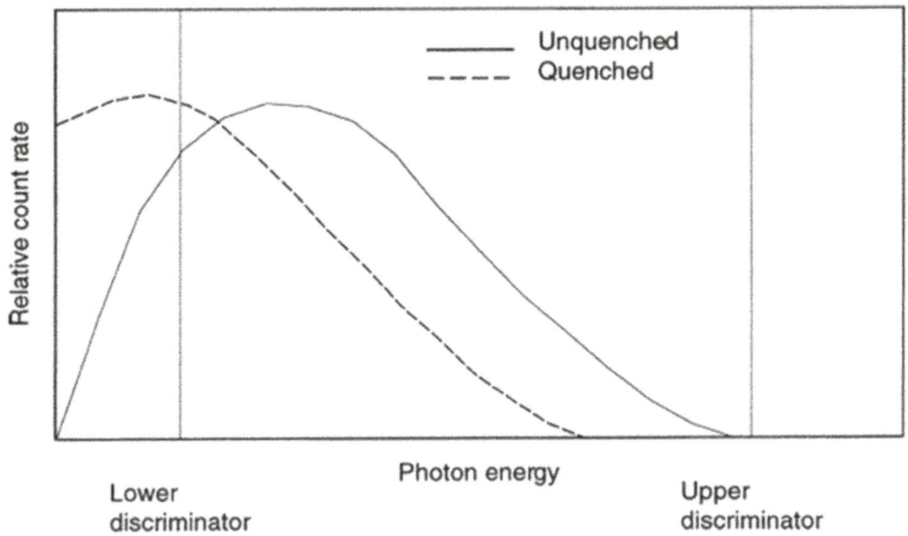

Figure 6.3. A typical beta particle spectrum obtained using a liquid scintillation counter for unquenched and quenched samples.

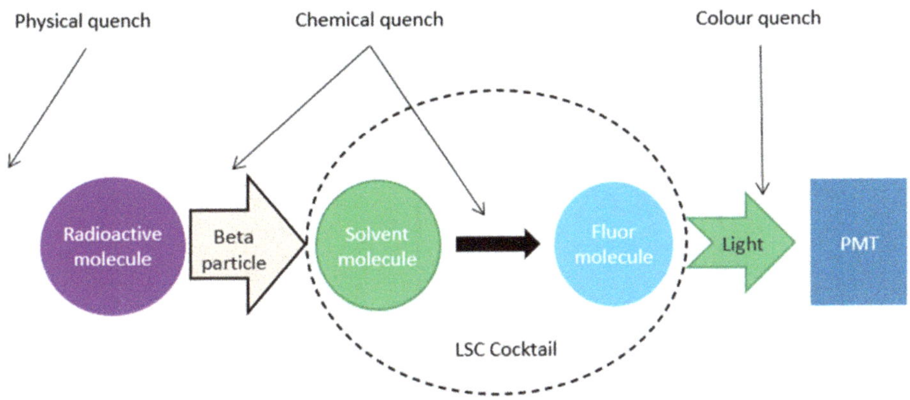

Figure 6.4. Quenching schematic (adapted from PerkinElmer Website 2020c).

3. Colour quenching due to the attenuation of light photons in the solution by substances (for example, blood) which absorb the emissions of either the primary or secondary scintillator; and
4. Dilution quenching, which may occur in samples of large volume due to a reduction in the concentrations of the scintillators, thereby decreasing scintillator output efficiency. Miniature vials containing cocktail volumes of down to 4 ml are often used to reduce this problem.

These quenching phenomena are schematically shown in figure 6.4 (adapted from PerkinElmer Website 2020b). There are several methods of quench correction (see section 6.9).

Quenching also affects background events originating within the cocktail, and this component is known as quenchable background. Background events originating outside the cocktail, however, are unquenchable; this type of event makes up around 70% of the total background.

6.3.2 Choice of vial

The choice of vial for liquid scintillation counting is affected by the volume, safety, the liquid scintillation cocktail chosen, chemical resistance, and performance. The vial wall also causes a reduction in the light reaching the PMT. Glass has excellent optical clarity and is typically chemically inert, but is fragile and therefore riskier from the perspective of radioactive contamination. Plastic tubes may hold static electricity (antistatic vials are available), but have reduced reflection for secondary scintillator light emissions compared to glass.

6.4 The detection of gamma emitters in liquid scintillators

The relatively low effective atomic number of organic liquid scintillators means that for the most commonly used gamma-emitting radionuclides, the gamma rays will interact principally by the Compton effect (figure 6.5), resulting in a scattered ray of lower energy and a recoil electron. The energy of the Compton electron will be converted into photons in exactly the same way as beta particles. A monoenergetic beam of gamma rays will produce a continuous spectrum of Compton electron

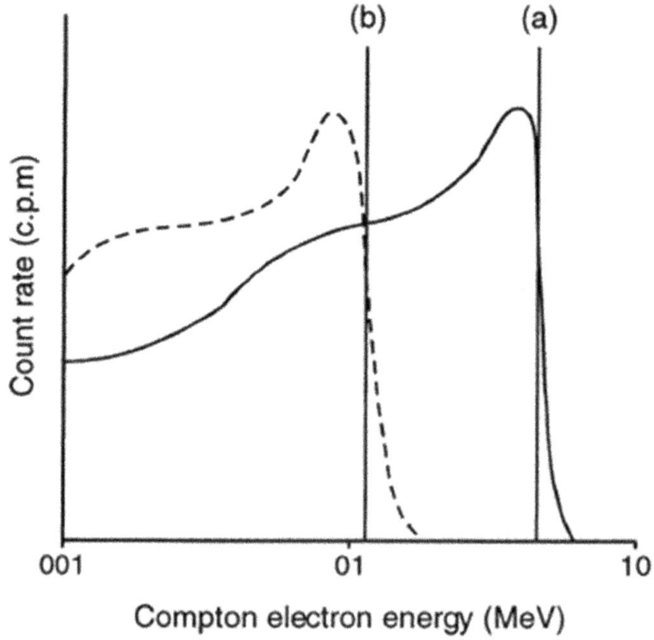

Figure 6.5. Compton spectra for ^{137}Cs obtained using a liquid scintillation counter, showing inflection points for (a) unquenched and (b) quenched samples.

energies (figure 6.5). Any quenching effects will alter the detected spectrum from a source of gamma rays in a similar manner to that for beta particles. A source of gamma rays may therefore be used to measure quenching (see section 6.8).

6.5 Liquid scintillation counting of electron-capture radionuclides

Radionuclides which decay by electron capture give rise to the emission of electrons. These may be either Auger electrons emitted in place of a characteristic x-ray, or internal conversion electrons produced in place of an associated gamma emission. These electrons are efficiently detected when counting electron capture radionuclides using a liquid scintillator. For example, only a small fraction of the x- and gamma-ray emissions from ^{125}I are absorbed by the scintillator and the spectrum is dominated by the Auger and conversion electrons. This results in detection efficiencies comparable with that of NaI(Tl) in its detection of the gamma emission. The counting efficiencies for three commonly used electron capture radionuclides are listed in table 6.1 and compared with those obtained using a well-type NaI(Tl) crystal. The disadvantages of using liquid scintillants for these radionuclides are the large increase in time spent preparing the samples and the expense of the scintillators.

6.6 Liquid scintillation cocktails

The liquid scintillation cocktail refers to the liquid medium which contains the sample during the analysis (L'Annunziata 2012), i.e. the combination of solvent, scintillator(s), sample, and any necessary additives such as surfactants (emulsifiers). Only cocktails used to measure activity in aqueous samples require surfactants. A good liquid scintillation cocktail benefits from having a good energy uptake from alpha and beta particles, low toxicity, a low concentration of ^{14}C, a high flash point, high quantum yield, high photon transmission, broad applicability, and an acceptable price (Edler 2015).

Cocktails can be either emulsifying (aqueous) if they contain an organic aromatic solvent, emulsifier, and scintillator or organic (nonaqueous/lipophilic) if they contain an organic aromatic solvent and a scintillator.

6.6.1 Solvents

The solvent makes up the bulk of the scintillation liquid cocktail, and most of the energy lost by the charged particles results in the ionisation and excitation of the

Table 6.1. Counting efficiencies for some commonly used electron capture radionuclides using a 76 mm long, 76 mm diameter well-type NaI(Tl) detector and a liquid scintillation counter.

Radionuclide	NaI(Tl) efficiency (%)	Liquid scintillation efficiency (%)
^{57}Co	90	65
^{125}I	82	76
^{51}Cr	7	30

solvent molecules. This energy is mainly dissipated as heat, but some is transferred to the scintillator, causing ionisation and excitation of its molecules. Good solvents must be efficient in converting and transferring energy. They should also be transparent to the photons emitted by the scintillators and provide adequate solubility for both scintillators and specimens.

Aromatic substances such as toluene or xylene have been historically used as solvents in 'classical' cocktails. Whilst effective at transferring energy, these organic solvents have proven to be extremely problematic due to their toxicity, high vapour pressure, flammability, strong smell, permeability thorough plastics, and disposal issues. This has led to the development of solvents for 'safer' cocktails with more favourable properties including higher flash points, low vapour pressure, low toxicity, low odour, and no permeation through plastics. Currently, the most popular of these solvents is di-isopropylnaphthalene (DIN) (Thomson 1991, L'Annunziata 2012), which has the additional advantage of being biodegradable, and is capable of handling relatively large proportions of water in solution. DIN is the solvent used in both Ultima Gold (PerkinElmer) and ProSafe+ (Meridian). Other cocktails use alternative solvents, such as: phenylxylylethane (PXE) in Scintisafe (Fisher), LumaSafe (PerkinElmer), and Ecoscint (National Diagnostics); and linear alkyl benzene (LAB) in Opti-Fluor and Emulsifier-Safe (PerkinElmer), Bio-Safe (RPI), Ecolume (ICN), and LumaSage (Lumac).

6.6.2 Scintillators

Scintillators convert the energy from alpha or beta particles into light energy. Ideally, scintillators should have a low sensitivity to quenching agents (section 6.3) and minimal overlap between the absorption and fluorescence emission spectra (referred to as a large Stokes shift). They also require sufficient solubility, a short fluorescence decay time, and high quantum yield (L'Annunziata 2012). The concentration of the scintillator(s) is generally a few grams per litre of solvent. Lower concentrations lead to poor counting efficiencies due to insufficient scintillator molecules to which the solvent may transfer its excitation energy. Higher concentrations of scintillator reduce counting efficiency by self-absorption.

There are usually two scintillators present in a liquid scintillation cocktail, referred to as the primary and secondary scintillators. The primary scintillator molecules absorb energy emitted from the radioactive source and decay with the emission of light photons; the emission is composed of a fast decay component (lifetime <80 ns) and a slower decay component (lifetime >300 ns). (Brooks 1979). The emission spectrum of good primary solutes, such as the commonly used PPO (2,5-diphenyloxazole), is generally in the UV and near-visible regions and does not perfectly match the peak spectral response of standard PMTs. PPO has good properties in terms of performance, purity, cost, and availability (L'Annunziata 2012).

Secondary scintillators (sometimes called wavelength shifters) absorb photons emitted by the primary scintillator and re-emit them at a lower energy which is better matched to the PMTs' photocathode response. The most popular current secondary scintillator is bis-MSB (1,4-bis(2-methylstyryl)benzene) because of its performance, solubility, purity, cost, and availability. bis-MSB is tending to replace the previously popular di-methyl POPOP, as it provides improved energy conversion in some applications (Passo and Cook 1994, L'Annunziata 2012). This results partly from its improved wavelength-shifting properties and partly through reducing the slow component of decay from the primary scintillator.

6.6.3 Additives/surfactants

Liquid scintillator solutions frequently contain additives to improve some aspect of their performance, such as the efficiency of energy transfer from solvent to scintillator. Radionuclides need close contact with the solvent to ensure efficient energy transfer. Solubilisers can assist in this, as they are chemical reagents which can break down a substance's macromolecular structure into subunits, thereby allowing them to be dissolved into a liquid scintillation cocktail (L'Annunziata 2012). Surfactants (emulsifiers) can be used for radioisotopes that are not miscible with aromatic solvents, but are not always required. They are only part of those cocktails which are designed for the uptake of aqueous solutions.

6.7 Sample preparation

The aim of sample preparation is to produce adequate dispersion of the sample in the liquid scintillator to allow for efficient energy transfer between the sample and the liquid scintillation cocktail with minimum quenching effects. This is a critical procedure in liquid scintillation counting if accurate and repeatable results are to be obtained. The subject of sample preparation has led to an extensive literature, and the reader is referred to some excellent review articles (Bransome 1970, Rapkin 1973, Peng 1977, L'Annunziata 2012). This section is intended to give only the briefest introduction to the more common methods available.

6.7.1 Homogeneous samples

Solubilisation

Biological samples are often considered challenging to prepare for liquid scintillation counting due to their components (such as colour or organic material) compared to those of other sample types. Many biological specimens, such as animal tissues, blood, urine, and amino acids, may be dissolved in liquid scintillators using chemical solubilisers (Thompson and Burns 2014). Solubilisation is the use of a chemical reagent to cause the breakdown (or digestion) of the macromolecular structure of interest, such that the smaller resulting subunits may dissolve directly into a liquid scintillation cocktail. Solubilisers are not compatible with all scintillators, and manufacturers frequently recommend their use with particular scintillators. The choice of base solvent is also important, as it not only acts as a vehicle for dissolving the sample/solubiliser and scintillator, but also carries the initial energy transfer from the nuclear decay. Solubilisers cannot dissolve all biological material or can sometimes only dissolve small amounts. In these cases, oxidation or combustion methods must be used.

Oxidation and combustion

Samples may be processed to prepare them for liquid scintillation counting by oxidation, frequently using nitric acid, or via combustion. Various combustion techniques have been described in the literature. This technique is applicable to almost any sample containing tritium, ^{14}C, or ^{35}S. Combustion in oxygen produces either $^{3}H_2O$, which can be collected as tritiated water, or the gaseous products $^{14}CO_2$ or $^{35}SO_2$, which may be trapped or absorbed by a suitable reagent and added into the scintillation cocktail. The benefit of complete combustion is that it removes issues due to colour quenching, self-absorption, and chemiluminescence (L'Annunziata 2012).

Commercial oxidisers are available. Operation is simple and ideal for large numbers of samples. However, equipment should be frequently cleaned and serviced, and the efficiency of sample recovery checked.

Gaseous absorption (e.g. breath tests)

Some radioactive gases may be soluble in the solvent and can be counted with little sample preparation. For example, the presence of the urease enzyme in *Helicobacter pylori* bacterium allows the conversion of ^{14}C-labelled urea into ^{14}C-labelled carbon dioxide, which may be detected in exhaled breath. Carbon dioxide may be trapped in a variety of bases. Both aqueous sodium hydroxide and alcoholic solutions of potassium hydroxide have been used for CO_2 sampling. However, inorganic bases generally have strong quenching characteristics and may produce severe chemiluminescence. It is therefore more appropriate to use organic bases such as hyamine hydroxide when collecting breath specimens from patients. ^{14}C breath tests used for this purpose have been superseded by a non-radioactive ^{13}C version of this test (Charest and Belair 2017).

6.7.2 Heterogeneous samples

Useful methods of counting aqueous or insoluble samples are in emulsions or suspensions or on solid supports. A fine dispersion of the sample in the scintillator is ideal for counting samples which are strong quenchers. Charged particles can escape from the phase boundary and react with the scintillator, while the quencher is confined to the aqueous phase and cannot therefore influence energy transfer in the scintillator. The applications of different counting configurations are:

1. Emulsion or colloid counting, which is used when it is essential to have a high capacity for dissolving water or aqueous samples;
2. Suspensions which can be used to count finely ground powders; and
3. Solid supports, such as filter papers or membranes immersed in a scintillator, which can be used to count, for example, chromatograms. This method can present problems, depending on the solubility of the sample. If elution from the support is slow, then the count rate will vary with time. The count rate may also be affected by the orientation of the support relative to the photomultiplier tubes.

6.7.3 Interfering processes

The method of preparing the sample for counting may result in the emission of photons which do not originate from the interaction of ionising radiation within the sample.

Chemiluminescence

Chemiluminescence is the emission of photons as a result of chemical reactions between any of the components of the counting mixture. It arises from the conversion of chemical energy into a molecular excitation, which undergoes radiative decay. The interaction of a charged particle with the scintillant produces a shower of photons in all directions within a few nanoseconds, whereas chemiluminescent events produce single photons only. Therefore, the use of multiple PMTs and coincident counting techniques, in which two or more PMTs are required to detect a signal in the same short time window, can significantly reduce the chemiluminescent count rates. This is because multiple photon events are preferentially detected, whilst single-photon events resulting from chemiluminescence are predominantly rejected. However, in the presence of significant chemiluminescence, this background can remain problematic, especially when sample count rates are relatively low. Here, multiple single-photon events occur within the same coincidence window.

To combat this, a short (~20 ns) delay can be set up between the signals in the PMTs, as described in section 6.10.1. This prevents true events being detected, whilst those from chemiluminescence will be, as the single-photon events are independent. If this delayed signal is subtracted from the true coincidence signal channel by channel in the MCA, the luminescence signal can be removed.

It is good practice to test samples with pH > 7 for chemiluminescence, as alkaline samples can cause a chemical reaction with the scintillation cocktail (L'Annunziata 2012). Although there are methods for measuring the chemiluminescent count rate of a radioactive sample (see section 6.10), it may be more satisfactory simply to test whether it is present and, if so, either to wait for it to decay (typically overnight) or to destroy it by further chemical treatment of the sample.

Phosphorescence

Phosphorescence is the result of photoactivation of the prepared sample by light. It differs from chemiluminescence in that the sample may be repeatedly photoactivated by exposure to light, whereas chemiluminescence is the once-only effect of a chemical reaction. Phosphorescence may be overcome by storing the sample in the dark. This is typically only required for an hour or two (L'Annunziata 2012).

Temperature control

Maintenance of the counting environment at a constant temperature improves the stability of the photomultiplier assemblies and is desirable at the location of the equipment. If the temperature is reduced to about −10 °C, improvements in the counting efficiency of some sample preparations (Rapkin 1968) and a reduction in chemiluminescence activity may result. However, solubility is also likely to be temperature dependent. The ability to run at low temperatures is not a common feature of counting equipment and may not be relevant in most cases.

6.8 Efficiency corrections for liquid scintillation counters

As described in section 6.3.1, the effect of quenching is to reduce the detected pulse height and shift the pulse height spectrum towards lower energies. Unless it is known for certain that the degree of quenching in a series of samples and standards is identical, it is essential to correct for differing counting efficiencies to standardise the results.

Several methods have been used to identify the extent of quenching and correct for its effect. These methods fall into four main categories: those using the samples alone by adding internal quench standards, using the samples alone and analysing the sample spectra, methods using external gamma sources, and efficiency tracing.

6.8.1 Internal standardisation

The earliest and simplest method is that of internal standardisation. The samples are counted once, so that an accurate counts per minute (CPM) value is recorded. A known and identical standard amount of the same radionuclide, which therefore always has the same decays per minute (DPM), is added to each sample (sometimes called 'spiking'). It is mixed well and the samples are recounted to obtain a new CPM. The volume of the spike must be small (e.g. 20 μl), or the quenching will be changed by dilution.

Let the initial count rate in the sample be S and the count rate after spiking be S'. If the activity in the 'spike' sample is T, then the counting efficiency E (i.e. count rate per activity) for this sample is given by:

$$E = \frac{(S' - S)}{T}.$$

The activity of the sample is therefore: S/E becquerels (Bq).

This method has several disadvantages:

1. The sample is spoilt, unless it is split in half, which is recommend for internal standardisation.
2. The count rate of the standard needs to be significantly larger than that of the sample (L'Annunziata 2012).
3. The activity of the standard must be accurately known (L'Annunziata 2012).
4. The spike must be in the same chemical form as the activity within the sample and must not alter the quenching of the sample significantly.
5. The method is very time-consuming, requires accurate sample transfer procedures, and cannot be automated.

However, internal standardisation is the only method which can provide an absolute measurement of quenching.

6.8.2 Sample channels ratio (SCR)

In addition to the normal counting channel A, a narrow channel, B, is set towards the lower-energy part of the pulse height spectrum (figure 6.6). The ratio of counts in A to counts in B is the sample channels ratio (SCR), which has a certain value for an unquenched sample. The effect of quenching is to reduce the count rate in channel A, and it can cause an increase or a smaller decrease in the counts in channel B. The SCR is therefore reduced by quenching and may be used as an index of quenching.

To use the SCR method, a number of standards containing equal activities are made up using the same scintillation cocktail as that used for the samples. The individual standards are quenched to differing degrees by adding different volumes of inactive sample material or specific quenching agent, leaving one standard unquenched. The standard and sample volumes should all be equal. The standards are counted under identical conditions to the samples and a 'quench correction curve' is plotted (figure 6.7). This shows counting efficiency relative to the unquenched standard versus SCR. The counting channels should be adjusted so that the efficiency falls monotonically with SCR, with only a gentle curve over the major part of its length. The activity in each of the samples relative to the standards

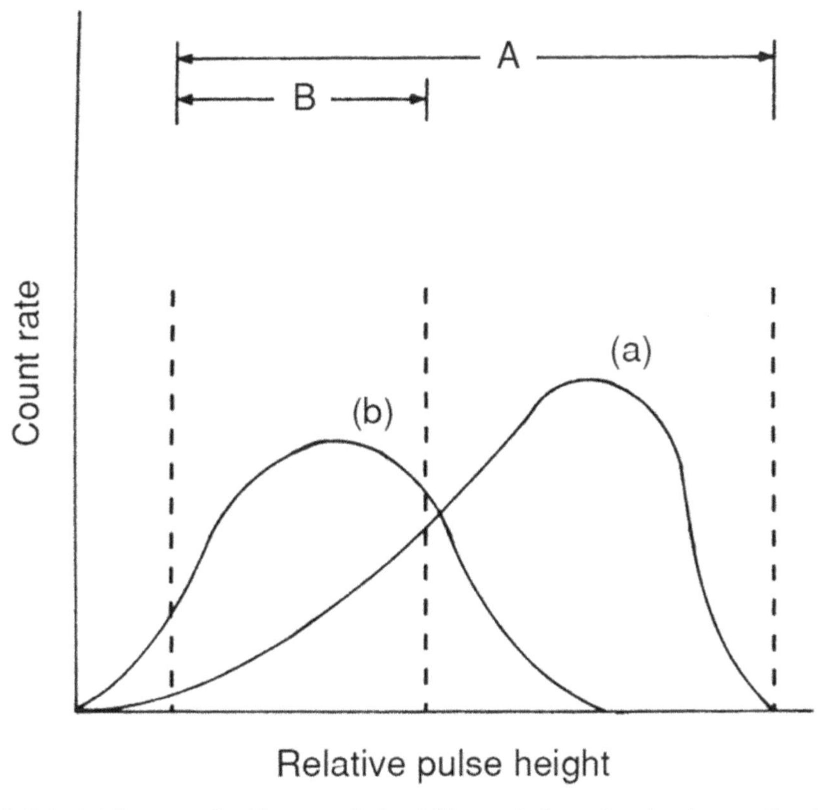

Figure 6.6. Pulse height spectra for (a) unquenched and (b) quenched samples, showing counting channels A and B for SCR measurements.

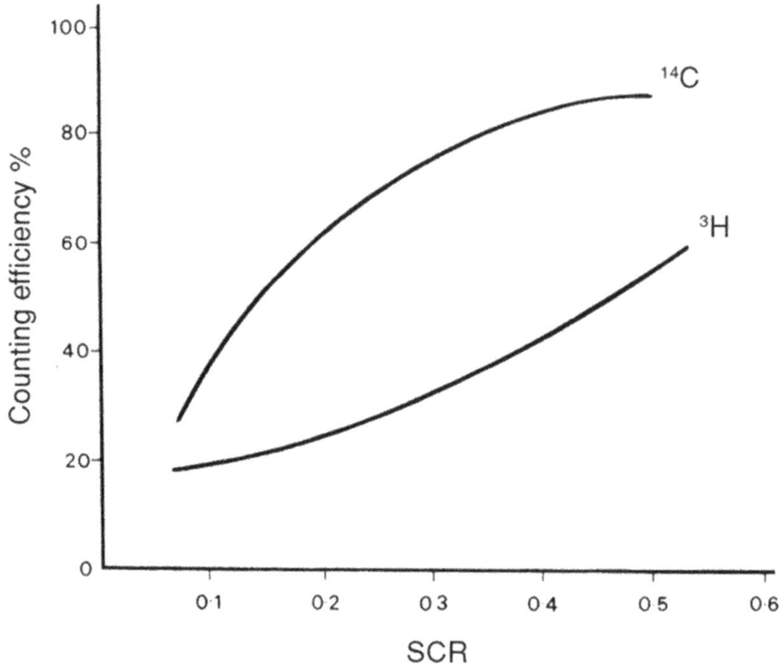

Figure 6.7. Quench correction curves obtained using the SCR method.

can then be found by reading off the relative counting efficiency for the observed sample's SCR and using this to correct the observed count rate.

The SCR has two main disadvantages. First, two counting channels are required for each radionuclide. In counters with preset channels only, the number of different radionuclides which can be counted in one run is halved. Second, the statistical precision of the measured SCR depends upon there being enough counts in both channels. With low-activity samples, or alternatively those that suffer from a high degree of quenching, this may result in very long counting times, especially in highly quenched samples.

6.8.3 Spectral index of sample (SIS)

The spectral index of a sample is based on the average energy of the beta energy spectrum, as plotted on a linear pulse height scale. It is defined by:

$$\mathrm{SIS} = K\frac{\sum_{x=0}^{u} Xn(X\chi)}{\sum_{x=0}^{u} n(X\chi)},$$

where:

SIS = spectral index

K = a constant relating to the maximum energy of the beta particle of the sample (L'Annunziata 2012).

$n(X)$ = number of counts with pulse heights between X and $X + \Delta X$
X = pulse height
u = upper limit of pulse height distribution

The shift in SIS due to quenching is independent of the sample volume and wall effects, as well as count rate, if the sample counts are large compared to the background. A correction curve of efficiency against SIS can be produced in the same way as for SCR. For the spectral index of a sample spectrum, the lower limit is set as low as possible, above the noise, and the upper limit is the top of the spectrum. As the whole spectrum is used, good statistical accuracy is available from quite low sample activities.

SIS is also relatively insensitive to structure in the spectrum, allowing quench correction of structured spectra, such as those obtained from ^{125}I, over a wider range of quench than is possible using more conventional channel ratios (section 6.8.1). The method depends on obtaining a high-resolution spectrum, which requires a wide dynamic range.

A parameter known as the spectral quench parameter of the isotope (SQP(I)), based on the channel number of the centre of gravity of the spectral distribution, may be used in an analogous way to the SIS method in instruments that incorporate an MCA with a logarithmic scale.

6.8.4 External standard channels ratio (ESCR)

Also known as external standardisation, this method relies on a high-activity gamma-emitting source that is external to the sample vial to provide an index of quenching. The external standard may be a few hundred kilobecquerels (kBq) of ^{133}Ba, ^{137}Cs, or ^{226}Ra. The external standard is brought close alongside or beneath each sample vial, with the result that its gamma radiation penetrates the sample, giving rise to recoil electrons following Compton scattering of the gamma radiation (section 6.4). These electrons interact with the scintillation cocktail in the same way as the sample beta radiation, and give rise to a broad pulse height spectrum which is also subject to the effects of quenching. During the sample count itself, the external standard is kept remote from the sample and very well shielded. Two special channels on the counter are usually reserved for counting the external standard spectrum. The ratio of counts in the upper of these to the lower is the ESCR, and gives an index of quenching in the same way as the SCR. However, since the external standard is the same no matter what radionuclide is being counted, the two special channels can be fixed to optimum settings to give a good relationship between relative efficiency and ESCR. These channels are preset by the manufacturer.

A second advantage of this method is that the external standard can be of sufficient activity to yield an ESCR with good statistical precision in a short time. However, unlike the SCR method, extra time is required for counting the external standard in addition to the sample counting time. Typically, 30 s is allowed for external standard counting, though this usually produces unnecessarily high precision. Alternatively, the external standard count may be terminated after, say,

10000 counts have been accumulated in one channel. The quench correction curve using ESCR as an index of quenching is generated in exactly the same way as for the SCR method, using a set of standards of varying quench.

Several problems can occur with the ESCR method. One of these arises when significant sample activity is detected in one of the ESCR counting channels. The ESCR is then found to vary with the sample activity in identically quenched samples. The first solution is to set the lowest ESCR channel to be higher than the maximum pulse height of the sample spectrum. This may be possible with tritium and ^{14}C samples, but not with higher-energy emitters. The best solution is to carry out a count of sample activity alone in the two ESCR channels and to use these values as backgrounds to be subtracted from the external standard counts for that sample. The first of these counts could be done at the same time as the actual sample count but, for reasons concerned with optimum window settings for quenched samples (section 6.10), the ESCR usually must be determined before the sample is counted. Thus, the time required to carry out the full ESCR determination is doubled, being one minute per sample in many cases.

The measured ESCR is usually sample volume independent over quite a range of sample volumes, but this should be checked for the particular instrument if widely differing sample volumes have to be used. Systems in which the external standard comes into position underneath the sample vial are likely to be better in this respect.

A problem sometimes occurs with the ESCR method when samples are kept in plastic vials for several hours before counting; this arises from the gradual diffusion of the cocktail scintillators into the vial wall. This causes the vial wall to act as a low-energy scintillator when irradiated by the external standard. Thus, the ESCR drifts downwards with time for constant quenching in the sample.

A further problem may be that only chemical and colour quenching are corrected. Losses due to the sample distribution of partially-soluble samples will not be accounted for.

Although it is generally an advantage to have fixed ESCR channels, it may be the case for highly quenched samples that the count rate in the upper channel is inadequate to give a sufficiently precise ESCR. It is often difficult for the user to readjust the ESCR channels to cope with this problem, as they are preset. This problem may be overcome by using an alternative scintillation cocktail.

6.8.5 Compton edge inflexion point (CEIP)

This technique was introduced for use with external standards which produce a well-defined Compton edge in the resulting scintillation spectrum (Long 1976). The position of the point of inflexion of the pulse height spectrum is used as an index of quenching. The effect of quenching is to shift the pulse height spectrum downwards and hence the position of the point of inflexion. A quench correction curve is set up in the same way as in the SCR and ESCR method, i.e. using variably quenched standards and plotting the relative efficiency versus the difference between the pulse heights of the CEIPs in the quenched samples and an unquenched sample. As this method relies on the top edge of the pulse height spectrum and not a ratio between high and low-energy portions, i.e. the shape of the spectrum, it claims some advantages over the ESCR method. It is less affected by sample activity, though with high-energy emitters, the Compton edge can be affected and correction is needed. The position of the Compton edge is also insensitive to sample volume and geometry and there is no impact due to the scintillator diffusing into the vial walls.

However, the CEIP method has been found to be rather less precise as an index of quenching, as the apparent position of the inflexion point is determined by the statistical errors of counting in narrow channels about this point. The channels ratio methods, which use the total count from wider windows, are more precise. The fact that CEIP looks only at the Compton edge position can also be a disadvantage. Changes in spectral shape, as may occur with optical quenching, can alter the efficiency of counting in a low-energy channel (such as for tritium) without having much impact on the CEIP. This makes it more important to use standards quenched in the same way and of the same density as the samples than may be the case with methods using more of the spectral information.

6.8.6 Mean pulse height calculations

The previously described spectral index parameter methods may also be applied to Compton spectra obtained from external irradiation of the sample. Quench may be indicated by shifts in the value of either the mean pulse heights or spectral end points. If a high-energy gamma emitter is used, it may be possible to ignore some of the lower channels corresponding to the typical emissions due to wall effect, hence eliminating errors due to solvent absorption into the walls of plastic vials. Again, mean pulse height analysis requires high-resolution linear energy spectra, but the use of the whole of the spectrum means that good statistical accuracy can be obtained in a relatively short external irradiation time. Spectral end point methods are typically used in instruments incorporating logarithmic counting channels.

6.8.7 Spectral analysis

Instead of using the plain Compton spectra generated by external gamma sources, liquid scintillation counters can utilise transformed spectra. The spectral distortions produced by artefacts such as wall effect, colour quenching, and variable volumes can be corrected for mathematically; in earlier methods, such distortions were eliminated from the analysis or were ignored, resulting in either a reduction in the dynamic range or reduction of the statistical accuracy. The external standard source needs to produce a Compton spectrum close to that of the most frequently used radionuclides (e.g. ^{133}Ba for ^{14}C counting) for maximum accuracy.

6.9 Implementation of quench correction

Quench correction in liquid scintillation counters can be implemented by storing the correction curve as a discrete set of variables such that the corresponding efficiency can be directly calculated for any reasonable value of quench index. Figure 6.8 provides a typical efficiency curve for ^{14}C. The simplest but least accurate method is to store a table of the discrete values of efficiency and quench index obtained from

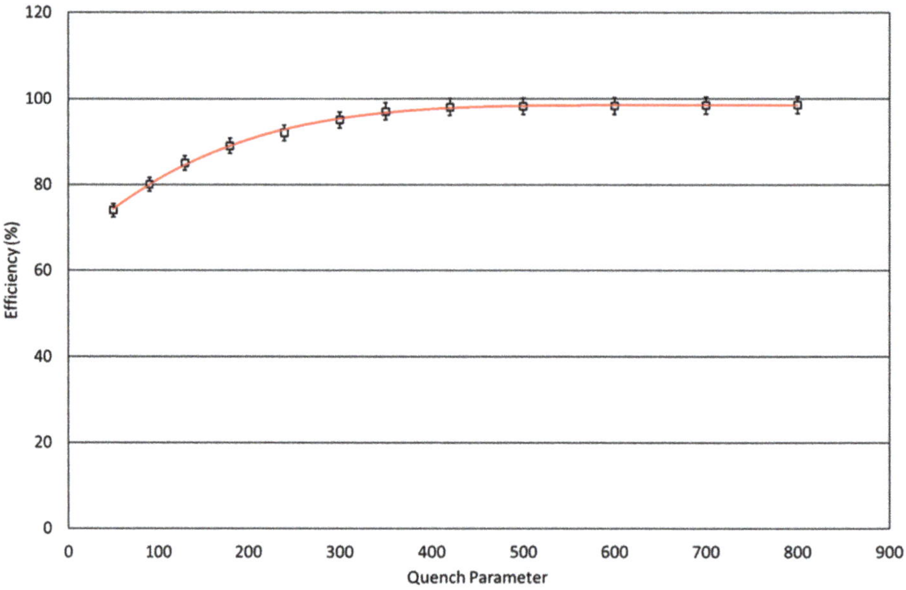

Figure 6.8. An example ^{14}C quench curve fitted with a third-order polynomial.

suitable standards. The efficiency corresponding to a particular sample quench index is obtained by linear interpolation between the pair of nearest points. Most counters, however, use the more satisfactory method of attempting to fit a continuous curve through the measured values obtained from the quenched standards.

6.9.1 Spline fitting

This method may be used to fit most relationships between two variables. No attempt is made to derive an analytic function that fits the whole curve, but segments of the curve are fitted by different functions of the same type, with mathematical constraints to ensure continuity between segments. This method can produce an excellent fit to any quench correction curve. Indeed, it can be too accurate, making the curve follow errors in individual points. To prevent this, the spline functions contain a smoothing parameter.

6.9.2 Polynomial fitting

A third-order polynomial is commonly found to be a good representation of the quench correction curve. The four parameters are deduced by a least-squares procedure. Although sharp changes in curvature cannot be accommodated, this fit is generally satisfactory in many applications.

6.9.3 Automatic efficiency correction

In the simplest counters with automatic efficiency correction, a polynomial curve is used with parameters determined by the user in a separate run of standards. These parameters are then entered into the program controlling the counting and processing of the samples.

Fully automatic counters can be programmed to use certain vials at the beginning of a batch as quenched standards and backgrounds, from which the parameters of the quench correction curves are derived and then stored to be used for processing of the unknowns. The user must input the absolute activity or the dose percentage for each standard. The results are presented in the same terms.

If conditions are sufficiently similar, it may be valid to use the same quench correction curves for more than one type of study.

Counters with automatic curve fitting often provide a graphical printout of the measured points and fitted curve for checking by the user. The option can also be provided to remove a point which is obviously in error and recalculate the fit.

Dual nuclide counting (see section 6.11) is handled in the same way, except that four quench correction curves (or three if it can be assumed that no low-energy nuclide is counted in the high-energy channel) have to be defined from sets of quenched standards of each nuclide in both channels. This does not pose a problem for a fully automated counter, but it is tedious if manual entry of curve constants is required. The method is described in section 6.11.

6.10 Chemiluminescence correction

The process of chemiluminescence was described in section 6.7.3. Although it is rarely necessary, the contribution of random chemiluminescent events to the observed count rate may be estimated by one of the following methods.

6.10.1 Correction by delayed coincidence

Correction for chemiluminescence can be performed by adding an additional fast coincidence channel, which imposes a fixed delay of about one microsecond on pulses from one of the photomultiplier tubes. The coincident pulses from beta interactions occur in a shorter time interval than this, so this channel will not detect true coincidences from the sample. However, the delay will not affect the rate of random coincidences that arise from chemiluminescent pulses which are coincident with each other or with beta interaction pulses. Thus, the usual counting channel will record the sum of true coincidences plus the random coincidences from chemiluminescence etc. and the delayed channel will count only the random coincidences. Subtraction of the two count rates gives the true sample count rate. The delayed coincidence channel must have an identical energy range to that of the main counting channel.

6.10.2 Correction by spectral analysis

If the counter acquires the full spectrum of each sample as it is counted, the chemiluminescent contribution is detectable as a sharp peak sitting on top of the low-energy portion of the beta spectrum. The computer can be programmed to slice off this peak, leaving an approximation to the correct sample spectrum, from which the count rate is calculated for the appropriate window settings. The counter may also indicate the presence of chemiluminescence on the printout and give some idea of its importance relative to the net sample count rate.

6.11 Dual nuclide beta counting

While the SCR method may be used for dual nuclide quench correction, the method is complicated and it is better to use one of the other methods.

One technique, usually referred to as the exclusion method, can be used when two samples with largely different beta particle energies are counted together. The analysers are set up with one counting channel for each nuclide, such that the lower edge of the high-energy channel is above the greatest pulse height produced by the low-energy nuclide in the least quenched sample (figure 6.9). Thus, the high-energy nuclide produces counts in both the high (H) and low (L) channels, while the low-energy nuclide counts only in channel L. However, for given activities, all three

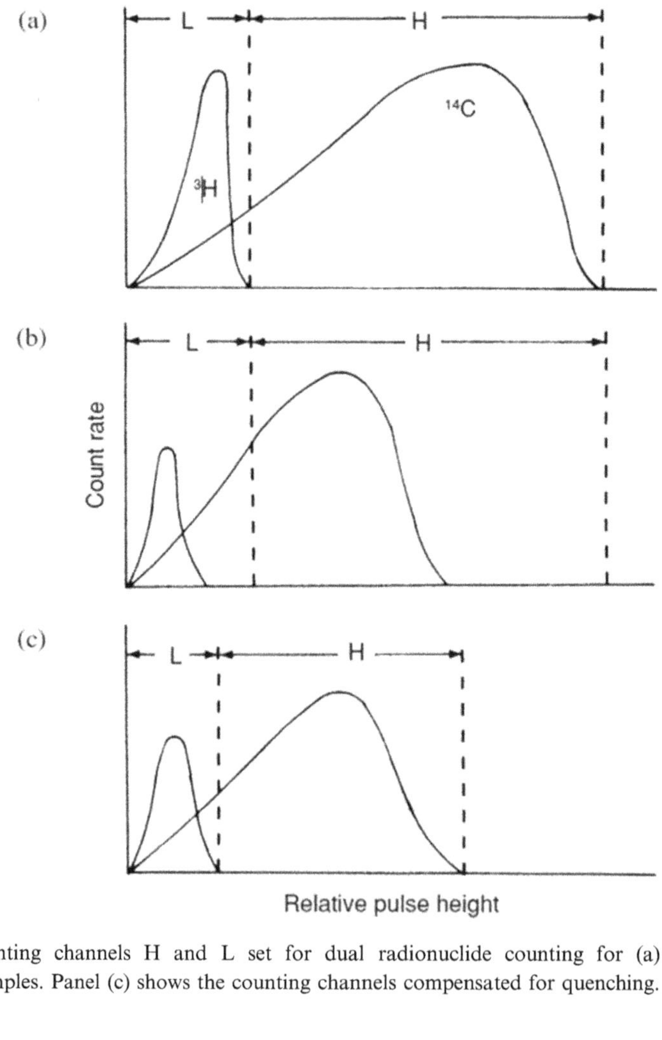

Figure 6.9. Counting channels H and L set for dual radionuclide counting for (a) unquenched and (b) quenched samples. Panel (c) shows the counting channels compensated for quenching.

count rates will depend on the degree of quenching. Whereas the activity of the high-energy nuclide is readily found using the methods described, it is necessary to extract the activity of the low-energy nuclide from the combination of low-energy activity, high-energy activity, and quenching which gives rise to the observed count in the low-energy channel.

Three quench correction curves are generated, using a set of variably quenched standards of each nuclide alone. These curves relate the ESCR or CEIP values to the relative counting efficiency of the high-energy nuclide in channel H (H/H), the high-energy nuclide in channel L (H/L), and the low-energy nuclide in channel L (L/L), respectively.

Analysis of a dual nuclide sample count after subtraction of the background count rates proceeds as follows (figure 6.10):

1. From the measured value of quench index, the efficiency, E_1, of counting the high-energy nuclide in its own channel is determined via point A on curve H/H. The high-energy count rate can then be converted into the absolute activity of the high-energy nuclide.
2. The efficiency, E_2, of counting the high-energy nuclide in the low-energy channel is found for the same value of quench index via point B on curve H/L. The previously determined high-energy nuclide activity multiplied by E_2

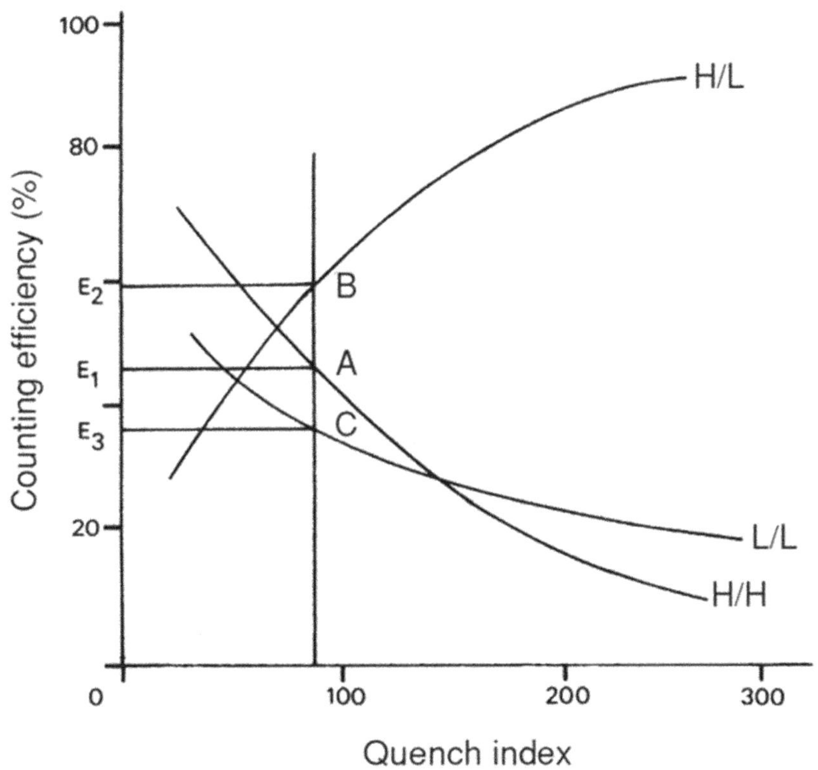

Figure 6.10. Quench correction curves for dual radionuclide counting.

gives the 'spillover' count rate into the low-energy channel, and this is subtracted from the total low-energy channel count rate.

3. The remainder is the count rate from the low-energy nuclide alone; this is converted to absolute activity using efficiency E_3, which is derived from the quench index value via point C on curve L/L.

In the inclusion method of dual radionuclide analysis, there is spill up in the pulse height spectrum of the lower-energy nuclide in the higher-energy channel. Here, a fourth quench curve is required that relates the quench index to the relative or absolute efficiency of the low-energy nuclide in channel H. As neither nuclide activity can be determined independently, the activities are obtained as the solutions of a pair of simultaneous equations that relate the total channel counts to efficiencies and activities.

Modern liquid scintillation counters can use more complex mathematical techniques to analyse the whole of the combined beta spectrum. Standard spectral indices of samples (SISs) for each radionuclide may be calculated for different quench levels. As the SIS of the combined spectrum is a combination of the SISs of the individual distributions and fractions of counts for each radionuclide, unknown count rates may be found if counting efficiencies are known for each radionuclide at a given quench level. These methods give maximum counting efficiencies without the need for spillover corrections. In order to be able to calculate counting rates over the entire quench range, efficiency curves must be stored for each radionuclide by counting a quenched series of reference standards plus the external standard Compton spectra if necessary.

6.12 Automatic quench compensation for beta counters

If fixed counting channels are used for a batch of samples for the same nuclides but widely varying quench, a problem can arise which seriously reduces the counting accuracy, especially in double-nuclide work. As quenching increases, the count rate of the high-energy nuclide in channel H falls, while its contribution to channel L ('spillover') rises (see figure 6.9(b)). This can have two consequences:

1. The count rate of the high-energy nuclide in channel H can fall to such an extent that a very long counting time is required to get sufficient statistical precision.
2. The spillover of the high-energy nuclide into channel L can swamp the count rate due to the low-energy nuclide, especially if the relative activity of the high-energy nuclide in the sample is much higher.

The situation is greatly improved by adjusting the upper edge of channel L and the lower edge of channel H to be just above the top of the quenched spectrum of the low-energy nuclide (figure 6.9(c)). In this way the counting efficiency of channel H is maximised without including any low-energy nuclide contribution and spillover is kept to a low level of <15 percent.

Modern systems may maintain optimal counting conditions by changing the discriminator levels so that the quenched spectrum is always kept within the counting region. This method is based on maximising the value of P/B, where P is the pulse height and B is the background count. With machines incorporating a multichannel analyser, a background spectrum is stored followed by the sample spectrum. Lower and upper limits for the regions are automatically adjusted to maximise the value of P/B for each sample. This method goes by the name of 'automatic window tracking', 'automatic quench compensation', 'spectral shift compensation', or 'automatic window setting', depending on the manufacturer of the machine.

Counts lost due to quenching are obviously not recovered, but the spillover of the high-energy radionuclide into the lower-energy counting channel is minimised. This quench-correcting method may be used in a counter without automatic quench compensation, but is quite time-consuming because of the need to count the background and sample for each new window setting.

6.13 Cerenkov counting

Liquid scintillation counters may also be used to count beta emitters by detecting Cerenkov radiation emission. This is electromagnetic radiation produced by a charged particle travelling faster than the velocity of light in the fluid (or glass/ plastic containers). A continuous spectrum is emitted in the wavelength band of about 300–700 nm (i.e. from the UV to the visible). This low-intensity light emission is highly directional, being confined to a cone around the direction of travel of the particle with a half-angle, θ, given by:

$$\cos\theta = \frac{1}{\beta n}$$

where β is the ratio of the velocity of the particle to the velocity of light in the medium and n the refractive index. βn must be greater than unity, and this defines a threshold particle energy below which Cerenkov radiation cannot be produced. In water, an organic solvent, or another similar clear liquid, this threshold is approximately 262 keV (L'Annunziata 2012), although a maximum energy of greater than 1 MeV is preferable for adequate light output.

Cerenkov radiation may be detected by a liquid scintillation counter, even in the absence of a scintillation cocktail. However, the anisotropic photon distribution reduces the probability of coincident detection by the two PMTs. This can be overcome by using a wavelength shifter which absorbs the Cerenkov radiation and re-emits isotropically at a longer wavelength, i.e. at a wavelength better matched to the PMT.

A number of beta-emitting radionuclides used in clinical applications produce Cerenkov radiation in aqueous solutions, examples being ^{32}P and ^{90}Y. The fact that a scintillator is not required results in an absence of chemical quenching but can still permit colour quenching. It should also be noted that only the portion of the beta particle spectrum above the threshold energy will be detected.

Counting efficiency for Cerenkov counting is affected by sample volume, chemical quenching agents (when cocktails are used), and colour quenching agents. The Cerenkov count rate is volume dependent, as the number of photons produced depends on the path length of the particles in the medium. The effects of colour quenching may be corrected by the methods described in section 6.8.

If an external standard is used, the Compton electrons should have sufficient energy to produce Cerenkov radiation. The higher the gamma-ray energy, the greater the proportion of the Compton electron spectrum which will produce Cerenkov radiation. This will produce a higher count rate per unit activity of an external standard. For this reason, ^{226}Ra, whose decay scheme includes gamma emissions with energies of up to 2448 keV is more suitable than ^{133}Ba (which has a maximum decay scheme gamma energy of 383 keV) or ^{137}Cs (with a maximum decay scheme energy of 662 keV) (Ekert and Ziegler Website 2020).

6.14 Quality control

Quality control for liquid scintillation counters depends on their intended use and local requirements. As a minimum, routine measurements of high- and low-energy long-lived check sources (such as ^{14}C and ^{3}H) are recommended in order to monitor system efficiency, along with a background measurement to observe changes in background conditions. The ^{14}C and ^{3}H measurements should be plotted on a range-control chart (section 3.5), as it is in the nature of PMTs to degrade over time. It is common for commercial systems to be provided with these check sources when purchased. Logging of the environmental conditions (temperature and humidity) is also recommended, as rapid changes can lead to measurement instability.

References

Birks J B 1964 *The Theory and Practice of Scintillation Counting* (Oxford: Elsevier)

Bransome E D 1970 *The Current Status of Liquid Scintillation Counting* (New York: Brune and Stratton)

Brooks F D 1979 Development of organic scintillators *Nucl. Instrum. Methods* **162** 477–505

Charest M and Belair M-A 2017 Comparison of Accuracy Between ^{13}C- and ^{14}C-Urea Breath Testing: Is an Indeterminate-Results Category Still Needed? *J. Nucl. Med. Technol.* **45** 87–90 Erratum in https://tech.snmjournals.org/content/45/4/316

Edler R 2015 *LSC Application Note: Cocktails for Liquid Scintillation Counting* PerkinElmer, Inc https://resources.perkinelmer.com/lab-solutions/resources/docs/APP_Cocktails-for-Liquid-Scintillation-Counting-011940_01.pdf

Ekert and Ziegler Website 2020 https://www.ezag.com/home/products/isotope_products/isotrak_-calibration_sources/downloads/nuclear_decay_schema_data/

Horrocks D L 1974 *Applications of Liquid Scintillation Counting* (Cambridge, MA: Academic Press)

Kozempel J, Mokhodoeva O and Vlk M 2018 Progress in targeted alpha-particle therapy. What we learned about recoils release from *in vivo* generators *Molecules* **23** 581

L'Annunziata M F (ed) 2012 *Handbook of Radioactivity Analysis* 3rd edn (Cambridge, MA: Academic Press) https://www.sciencedirect.com/book/9780123848734/handbook-of-radioactivity-analysis

Long E C 1976 Liquid Scintillation Counting Theory and Techniques (Beckman Technical Publication 915-NUC-76-7.T)

Passo C J and Cook G T 1994 *Handbook of Environmental Liquid Scintillation* (Meriden, CT: Packard Instrument Company) https://www.perkinelmer.com/CMSResources/Images/44-73395BKT_LSCHandbookEnvironmentalLiquidScintillationSpectrometry.pdf

Peng C T 1977 *Sample Preparation in Liquid Scintillation Counting* Review 17 (Arlington Heights, IL: Amersham Corporation) The Radiochemical Centre

Peng C-T, Horrocks D L and Alpen E (ed) 1980 *Liquid Scintillation Counting, Recent Applications and Development* vol 2 (Cambridge, MA: Academic Press)

PerkinElmer Website 2020a https://www.perkinelmer.com/uk/lab-prducts-and-services/application-support-knowledgebase/radiometric/alpha-beta.html

PerkinElmer Website 2020b (https://www.perkinelmer.com/uk/lab-products-and-services/application-support-knowledgebase/radiometric/quench.html

PerkinElmer Website 2020c https://www.perkinelmer.com/uk/lab-products-and-services/application-support-knowledgebase/radiometric/liquid-scintillation-counting.html

Rapkin E 1968 Temperature Control in Liquid Scintillation Counting (Intertechnique Technical Review)

Rapkin E 1973 Preparation of Samples for Liquid Scintillation Counting by Combustion (Intertechnique Technical Review)

Ross H, Noakes J and Spaulding J 1991 *Liquid Scintillation Counting and Organic Scintillators* (Boca Raton, FL: CRC Press)

Thomson J 1991 Di-isopropylnaphthalene—a new solvent for liquid scintillation counting *Liquid Scintillation Counting and Organic Scintillators* ed H Ross, J E Noakes and J Spaulding (Boca Raton, FL: Lewis Publishers) 19–34

Thompson J and Burns D A 2014 *Liquid Scintillation Application Note: LSC Sample Preparation and Counting of Biological Samples* PerkinElmer https://resources.perkinelmer.com/lab-solutions/resources/docs/APP_BiologicalSamplePrepAndCounting.pdf

IOP Publishing

Radioactive Sample Counting: Principles and Practice
(Second Edition)
IPEM report 85
Sofia Michopoulou

Chapter 7

Automatic blood sampling systems (ABSSs)

Lucy Pike

7.1 Introduction to ABSS instrumentation

To generate accurate information about the kinetics of an injected radiotracer, patients are injected on the scanner couch and fast dynamic PET or SPECT acquisitions are performed as the tracer enters the bloodstream and is distributed into the organs and tissues. The measured uptakes in the reconstructed images are compared to model predictions by convolving the tracer concentration in arterial blood or plasma (the input function) with specific model functions (Eriksson *et al* 1988). The most accurate method for obtaining the input function is to perform arterial blood sampling. Manual sampling can be performed with the blood samples counted in a gamma counter; however, this is difficult as samples need to be drawn rapidly over the first few minutes of the study to ensure that the peak of the input function is captured. To reduce the requirement for manual sampling, automatic blood sampling systems (ABSSs) have been designed that facilitate measurements with high temporal resolution; such systems also have the advantage of reducing the radiation dose to staff.

The general principle of an ABSS is straightforward; however, setting the system up can be very complicated. Figure 7.1 shows a schematic diagram of an ABSS.

A peristaltic pump draws the blood from the arterial catheter at a constant rate through the detector. The detector is connected to a PC running software that continually logs the counts from the detector with a timestamp. A three-way tap is integrated into the tubing after the detector to allow for the withdrawal of manual samples. Finally, the withdrawn blood is collected in a blood bag for storage and disposal.

7.2 ABSS types

Due to the fact that arterial blood sampling in PET studies is invasive and complex, it is limited to a small number of centres that perform specialist research studies. As such, there are limited options for purchase of 'off the shelf' ABSSs, particularly for human studies.

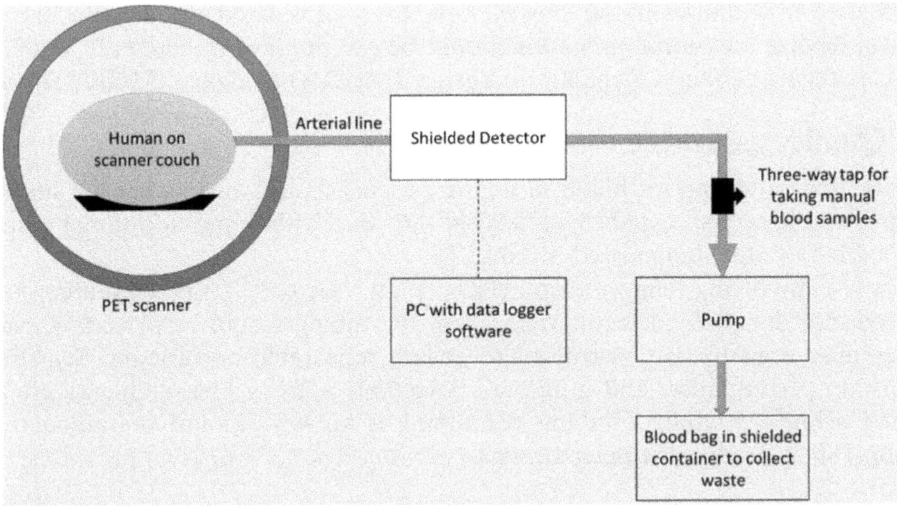

Figure 7.1. Schematic diagram of an automatic blood sampling system (ABSS) connected to a human.

There are two general types of detector design. Some systems use a single detector unit only, allowing counting in singles mode. This tends to have a higher sensitivity, but suffers from greater noise from external sources.

More recent designs incorporate two detector units for counting in coincidence, thus reducing the amount of scatter measured, but offering lower sensitivity. These two-detector systems may allow counting in both singles mode and coincidence mode, which makes them compatible for both SPECT and PET tracers.

The selection of an ABSS will therefore mainly be determined by the scope of the intended work (the use of SPECT and/or PET tracers, PET-CT, or PET-MR). Further key performance factors to consider are sensitivity, the signal-to-noise ratio, stability, and count-rate performance, all of which will be determined by the type and size of the detector and amount/type of radiation shielding.

7.3 Specification and purchase of an ABSS

If PET-CT is the only application, the equipment (detector, pump, PC, and waste storage) can conveniently be set up on a shielded trolley that can be wheeled into the scanning room as and when required. For PET-MR, this is not currently feasible, since the different components are not all MR compatible. In addition, all currently available commercial systems use PMTs, which need to be kept outside the scanning room as they are heavily affected by the magnetic field (Breuer *et al* 2010). Therefore, consideration needs to be made for running light guides outside the scanning room to the PMTs and PC. Some groups have been developing blood sampling systems using silicon photomultipliers (SiPMs) (Velasco *et al* 2019) and avalanche photodiodes (APDs) (Breuer *et al* 2007) for PET-MR applications; however, these have not been approved for human use. The peristaltic pump may not be MR compatible, either. In place of this, an MR-compatible infusion pump can be used to withdraw blood; however, as this is considered an 'off-label' use of a medical device, additional processes should be put in place in line with Medicines and Healthcare products Regulatory Agency (MHRA) guidance (MHRA 2014).

7.4 Quality assurance

Quality control testing for blood sampling systems should mirror that for standard gamma counters, as described in section 4.6, but with some additional tests as detailed below and summarised in table 7.1.

For tests involving long-lived sources, a small ^{68}Ge or ^{137}Cs point source should be used that fits in the detector well where the tubing would be placed. A plastic holder may need to be constructed to ensure repeatable positioning. Sensitivity, count-rate performance, and minimum detectable activity measurements are performed using a section of tubing containing a known amount of radioactivity, usually 18F, placed in the detector well.

Table 7.1. Recommended quality control tests and frequencies for automatic blood sampling systems.

Test	Suggested frequency
Cleaning and decontamination	Daily/weekly, depending on use
Functional checks	Prior to counting session
Background checks	Baseline measured at commissioning and prior to counting session
Sensitivity or efficiency	Baseline measured at commissioning, annually, and after any repairs
Constancy and long-term stability	Tolerances set at commissioning or after major upgrade; constancy of sensitivity is measured prior to counting session, and long-term stability is assessed quarterly
Energy resolution and photopeak channels	Checked prior to counting session; recalibration performed as part of detector normalisation
Normalisation	At commissioning and quarterly (unless otherwise specified by the manufacturer)
Cross-calibration	Not required if manual samples are used to calibrate the blood curve on a per-patient basis; if not, perform straight after the PET (or SPECT) cross-calibration
Repeatability	At commissioning
Shielding and background characterisation	At commissioning; will be dependent on the location of the detector in the scanner room and the amount and distribution of radioactivity in the patient
Decay correction	At commissioning
Count-rate performance	At commissioning
Minimum detectable activity	At commissioning
Adsorption and dispersion effects	Perform at commissioning for each isotope, type, and length of tubing to be used; repeat before new tubing is used
MR interference	At commissioning
Database management	Quarterly/annually, depending on use

7.4.1 Minimum detectable activity

In addition to the higher activity limit for the detector, it is useful to determine the lower detection limit. The minimum detectable activity (MDA) is the minimum amount of activity that yields the detection limit and is calculated as follows:

$$\text{MDA} = \frac{N_T - N_B}{f\epsilon VT},$$

where N_T is the total counts for the sample plus background, N_B is the background counts, f is the radiation yield per disintegration for the specific isotope, ϵ is the sensitivity, V is the sample volume, and T is the sample counting time (Knoll 2000, Roehrbacher 2015).

7.4.2 Adsorption

Some radiotracers are very lipophilic and can have high adsorption on the inner walls of the tubing, resulting in an artificially high background count. This will be dependent on the tubing material used and the manufacturer should provide details of appropriate tubing compatible with the pump. If no data on adsorption properties is provided for the radiotracer and tubing combination to be used and there is no information in the literature, users should check for adsorption, as this can have a significant effect on the arterial input function. To check for adsorption, a solution of the radiotracer should be passed through the ABSS. If adsorption occurs, a gradual increase in the activity concentration will be seen over time and radioactivity will remain even after emptying the system.

7.4.3 Dispersion effects

Since the arterial blood sample is transported to the detector via a length of tubing outside the body, there is a delay in the measurement. The concentration also spreads out as it passes along the tubing. This is known as dispersion and needs to be corrected for in kinetic modelling. The degree of dispersion will depend upon the length of tubing used and the viscosity of the radiotracer. To correct for this, the step function (figure 7.2) needs to be measured using blood samples with and without radiotracer present, as described by Munk *et al* (Munk 2008).

7.4.4 MR interference

For systems used in PET-MR, additional consideration needs to be given to the compatibility of the blood sampling system with the MR scanner. Potential interference in the measured signal may arise from electromagnetic radiation in the radiofrequency range or signals at the resonant frequency of the MR scanner (Breuer *et al* 2010). To test for any interference, measurements of the sensitivity and energy resolution should be made outside the MR room as a reference and then repeated in the MR room while typical MR sequences are run.

The presence of the ABSS may also introduce artefacts into the MR image. Tests for noise and geometric distortion in the images should be performed using standard MR phantoms with and without the ABSS present.

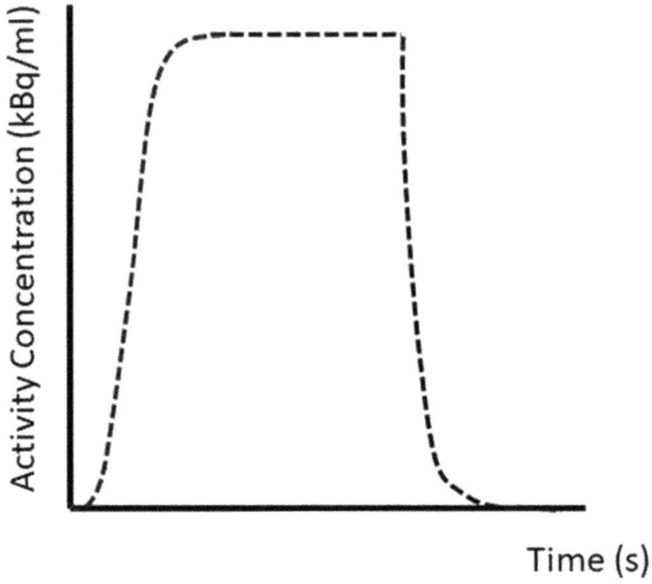

Figure 7.2. Schematic diagram of a dispersion curve for an ABSS.

7.4.5 Pump tests

A full description of the maintenance, routine testing, and commissioning of the pump is beyond the scope of this document. Users should seek advice from the device manufacturer and medical engineers with experience in the routine testing of similar devices.

Testing will typically cover visual checks, pressure and rate checks, electrical safety checks, and emergency alarms/stop functions.

References

Breuer J *et al* 2007 MR-compatible blood sampler for PET *2007 IEEE Nuclear Science Symp. Conf. Record* 5 (Manhattan, NY: IEEE) 3426–29

Breuer J *et al* 2010 Evaluation of an MR-compatible blood sampler for PET *Phys. Med. Biol.* **55** 5883–893

Eriksson L *et al* 1988 Automated blood sampling systems for positron emission tomography *IEEE Trans. Nucl. Sci.* **35** 703–07

Knoll G 2000 *Radiation Detection and Measurement* 3rd edn (New York: Wiley)

MHRA 2014 Guidance for off-label use of a medical device (Medicines and Healthcare Products Regulatory Agency) https://www.gov.uk/government/publications/medical-devices-off-label-use/off-label-use-of-a-medical-device

Munk O L, Keiding S and Bass L 2008 A method to estimate dispersion in sampling catheters and to calculate dispersion-free blood time-activity curves *Med. Phys.* **35** 3471–81

Roehrbacher F, Bankstahl J P, Bankstahl M, Wanek T, Stanek J and Sauberer M *et al* 2015 Development and performance test of an online blood sampling system for determination of the arterial input function in rats. *EJNMMI Phys.* **2** 1

Velasco C *et al* 2019 Development of a blood sample detector for multi-tracer positron emission tomography using gamma spectroscopy. *EJNMMI Phys* **6** 25

IOP Publishing

Radioactive Sample Counting: Principles and Practice (Second Edition)
IPEM report 85
Sofia Michopoulou

Chapter 8

Uncertainties in measurements from radioactivity sample counters

Peter O'Sullivan

8.1 Introduction

The process of taking any measurement will always include an inherent uncertainty, and so a complete description of any measurement should always include an assessment of this uncertainty. This uncertainty value can indicate the quality of the measurement and the confidence with which it can be used.

The measurement of counts detected from a radioactive sample is subject to both random and systematic errors. Random errors include the unavoidable uncertainty in a result which arises from the random nature of radioactive decay. Systematic errors, e.g. the volume or mass of a sample, can usually be optimised by a careful and thoughtful methodology and the use of appropriate apparatus.

The ultimate purpose of this assessment is to be able to define the uncertainty in our clinical or scientific parameter, e.g. glomerular filtration rate measurement or leak-testing result.

8.2 Inherent errors

Owing to the nature of the process of radioactive decay, it is impossible to state exactly when an atomic nucleus will disintegrate. However, this randomness is not unbounded.

For any radionuclide, there is a fixed probability that disintegration will occur within a fixed time. This means that when many atoms are considered instead of a single atom, repeated measurements of the number disintegrating within a given time are not equal, but are clustered around a most probable value.

If the measurement time is small and the count rate is low, the probable number of counts detected will also be small and the distribution of counts obtained will follow a Poisson distribution. As the mean count, N, increases, the distribution of

doi:10.1088/978-0-7503-3895-0ch8

counts approximates to a Gaussian (or normal) distribution with a mean N and a standard deviation $\sqrt{N}$. The Gaussian distribution is a symmetrical bell-shaped curve for which 68.3% of the area under the curve (or the same percentage of the total number of measurements) falls between ±1 standard deviation from the mean. Similarly, 95.5% of observations fall between ±2 standard deviations, and 99.7% fall between ±3 standard deviations from the mean.

In practice, a sample is only counted once, or possibly twice. Although the precise relationship of this count to the mean of the distribution curve is not known, it can be assumed that there is a 99.7% probability that the count is within ±3 standard deviations of the mean. Therefore, it is reasonable to use the count obtained as the best estimate of the mean and assign it a standard error equal to the square root of the count, since this is the best estimate of the standard deviation of the underlying distribution.

The percentage or relative standard deviation (ν_N) is the standard deviation (σ_N) expressed as a percentage of the mean. This is also known as the coefficient of variation.

We can apply the same definition to the percentage standard error of the count. The percentage standard error and standard error are assigned the same symbols as the corresponding deviation. If N counts are obtained in a time T, $\nu_N = 100\sigma_N/N$ or, since $\sigma_N = \sqrt{N}$, $\nu_N = 100/\sqrt{N}$. By counting the same sample for $2T$, $2N$ counts will be obtained, giving a percentage standard error of $100/2\sqrt{N}$. The precision of the measurement is therefore increased, corresponding to a $1/\sqrt{2}$ reduction in ν_N. In practice, it is rarely necessary to reduce the percentage standard error below 1%, as other errors in laboratory procedure are likely to be more significant. A count of 10 000 gives a percentage standard error of 1%.

The standard error of the mean of any number of single counts is essentially the same as the standard error of a single count of equal total time. However, multiple counts give a check on the stability of the counter and reproducibility of the readout device. If computer analysis is to be performed, it could easily be arranged that if two counts do not lie, for example, within ±3σ of each other, that they are rejected or at least attention is drawn to a possible error.

A useful way of checking a counter manually is to count a sample or standard ten times to ensure that on average 6–7 of the results fall within ±1 square root of the mean. If a count N is obtained in time T, then the count rate, n, is given by

$n = \frac{N}{T}$, hence $\sigma_n = \frac{\sqrt{N}}{T} = \sqrt{\frac{n}{T}}$, where σ_n is the standard error of the count rate.

8.3 Error propagation

The counting statistics form one part of the total uncertainty of a measurement. To calculate the overall uncertainty, we must take account of the uncertainties which are generated in the production of the sample. The actual sources of uncertainty will vary depending on the method of production, but will typically include the uncertainties of the total volume of the standard and measured aliquot and the weight or activity measurement of the radiopharmaceutical vial/syringe.

If one has measurements $x,\ldots,z$ with associated uncertainties $\delta x,\ldots, \delta z$, and these are used to compute the function $f(x,\ldots, z)$, as long as the uncertainties are independent and random, then the uncertainty in f is:

$$\delta f = \sqrt{\left(\frac{\partial f}{\partial x}\delta x\right)^2 + \ldots + \left(\frac{\partial f}{\partial z}\delta z\right)^2}\,.$$

This expression can be simplified into the two familiar expressions for the uncertainty in sums and differences and into the uncertainties in products and quotients.

The uncertainty in sums and differences

If one has measurements $x,\ldots,z$ with associated uncertainties $\delta x,\ldots, \delta z$, and these are used to compute

$$f = x + \ldots + z - (u + \ldots + w),$$

if the uncertainties in $x,\ldots,w$ are known to be independent and random, then the uncertainty is the quadratic sum

$$\delta f = \sqrt{(\delta x)^2 + \ldots + (\delta z)^2 + (\delta u)^2 + \ldots + (\delta w)^2}\,.$$

However, if these measurements are not independent, we can estimate the uncertainty using this expression:

$$\delta f \approx \delta x + \ldots + \delta z + \delta u + \ldots + \delta w.$$

The uncertainty in products and quotients

If one has measurements $x,\ldots,z$ with associated uncertainties $\delta x,\ldots, \delta z$, and these are used to compute

$$f = \frac{x \times \ldots \times z}{u \times \ldots \times w},$$

if the uncertainties in $x,\ldots,w$ are known to be independent and random, then the uncertainty in f is the sum in quadrature of the original fractional uncertainties:

$$\frac{\delta f}{|f|} = \sqrt{\left(\frac{\delta x}{x}\right)^2 + \ldots + \left(\frac{\delta z}{z}\right)^2 + \left(\frac{\delta u}{u}\right)^2 + \ldots + \left(\frac{\delta w}{w}\right)^2}\,.$$

Again, if the measurements are not independent, we can estimate the uncertainty using this expression:

$$\frac{\delta f}{|f|} \approx \frac{\delta x}{|x|} + \ldots + \frac{\delta z}{|z|} + \frac{\delta u}{|u|} + \ldots + \frac{\delta w}{|w|}.$$

8.4 Errors due to background counts

Unwanted counts due to background radiation or electronic noise cannot be eliminated completely. These background counts will increase the error in the desired result above that described in the previous section. The standard error of the difference (or sum) of two count rates is found using the relationship:

$$\sigma_{1 \neq 2} = \sqrt{\sigma_1^2 + \sigma_2^2}.$$

Hence

$$\sigma_S = \sqrt{\frac{n_{S+B}}{T_{S+B}} + \frac{n_B}{T_B}},$$

where:

σ_S = the standard error of the background corrected sample count rate,
n_{S+B} = the count rate from the sample (including background),
n_B = the background count rate,
T_{S+B} = the time for which the sample (including background) was counted, and
T_B = the time for which the background was counted.

If the sample count rate is much higher than the background, only a crude estimate of the background is needed. For example, if the sample count is 10 000 and the background for the same time is 10, then the latter is much smaller than the standard error of the sample count. Conversely, if the two are similar, then they must be counted for almost equal times (and much longer overall). The optimal division of the total counting time for the sample and the background is given by Wagner *et al* (1968):

$$\frac{T_{S+B}}{T_B} = \sqrt{\frac{n_{S+B}}{n_B}}.$$

The value of the background count and the time available places a lower limit on the activity which can be measured with a given degree of accuracy. For example, if the background count rate is 10 cpm (counts per minute) and the sample plus background is 20 cpm, then it would be necessary to count the background for 100 min and the sample for 150 min (approximately the correct ratio of times) to give an answer within ±10% with 95% confidence.

8.5 The use of standards

Usually, when performing measurements of radioactivity, one count is compared to another, often that of a standard. This introduces another error and, in order to calculate it, the percentage standard error must be used. The error connected with the product or quotient of two counts is found using the relationship:

$$v_m = \sqrt{v_1^2 + v_2^2},$$

where m = the product or division of v_1 and v_2.
v_m = the percentage or relative standard deviation.

In this case, the optimum division of total counting time can be shown to be given by:

$$\frac{T_1}{T_2} = \sqrt{\frac{n_2}{n_1}}.$$

It will be noted that this is the inverse of the relation obtained for the sum or difference of two counts and means that the higher-activity standard can be counted for a shorter time than the lower-activity sample.

The probable statistical error involved in any radioactive measurement, together with the optimum counting times, can be calculated from the above considerations and it is important to bear these in mind when creating a protocol for an application so that errors may be minimised while, at the same time, not wasting counting time. Generally, counting times are chosen such that the errors in the standard and any typical or important sample are kept below the required level, often 1%. A typical protocol would be to count each item for at least 10 000 counts or 10 min, whichever comes first.

8.6 Other uncertainties in counting samples

The counting statistics form one part of the total uncertainty of a measured sample. To calculate the overall uncertainty, we must take account of the uncertainties which are generated in the production of the sample. The actual sources of uncertainty will vary, depending on the method of production, but will typically include the uncertainties of the total volume of the standard and measured aliquot and the weight or activity measurement of the radiopharmaceutical vial/syringe.

Systematic and random uncertainties

It is important to be aware of the possible sources of systematic error in standards and eliminate them where possible. For systematic uncertainties that cannot be eliminated, it is important to find a way to estimate their magnitude, and then to combine it in quadrature with the random uncertainties to find the total uncertainty:

$$\delta f = \sqrt{\left(\delta f_{Ran}\right)^2 + \left(\delta f_{sys}\right)^2}.$$

The use of simulation for error propagation

Propagating uncertainties for a clinical test, such as the glomerular filtration rate, can become quite complex; see section 10.3. An alternative method is the use of simulation, which is a powerful tool for combining uncertainties from many sources. A recent publication by Holness *et al* showed similar results to those presented in section 10.3 using this method.

Reference

Wagner H N Jr, Walton W W and Jacquez J 1968 *Principles of Nuclear Medicine* ed H N Wagner Jr 1 (London: WB Saunders & Co.) 3

Chapter 9

Data analysis

Sofia Michopoulou

9.1 Basic data

The basic information obtained for a sample by a liquid scintillation or gamma counter consists of the sample's identification, the time for which it was counted, the separate gross counts recorded in each counting channel (or energy window), and the time of day at which the counts were recorded. From this, most counters calculate the count rate in each channel and the associated statistical error. Some systems also have in-built sensitivity factors and provide the activity of the measured isotope as part of their basic data output. Current gamma counting systems also provide the gamma spectrum for further review and analysis, but in some cases, the purchase of an additional software license is required to enable the spectrum to be exported. Liquid scintillation counters will also normally derive the quenching index. In the field of sample counting, a traditional term for any calculation performed on the basic information is 'data reduction'.

9.2 Data handling

Automatic sample counters have been commercially available since the 1960s and have proved to be extremely reliable machines. One consequence of this is that there are a profusion of data-handling systems, incorporated or attached to them, that are still in everyday use.

The simplest allow basic counting parameters to be set and can output the count data to a PC. Current sample counters have integral computing facilities and networking capabilities, such as LAN connectivity. Common types of data handling are described in this chapter. In addition to hardware, any data-handling software provided by the manufacturer needs to be CE marked. When in-house software is to be used for further data handing to help inform clinical decisions, such software should be developed within a quality management system that complies with the Medical Devices Regulations (The Medical Devices Regulations 2002).

doi:10.1088/978-0-7503-3895-0ch9

9.3 Background subtraction

Background counts impact the counting accuracy of sample counters; therefore, background subtraction methods are routinely required. Background counts can vary with time due to drift in the gain of the PM tube, variations in the cosmic radiation background, local changes in radiation levels, or changes in detector temperature and should be checked regularly.

Current counting systems calculate the background count rate or allow the user to enter a preset background count rate for each counting channel. When the sample count rates are computed, these values are automatically subtracted to give the net count rates for each channel. The background count rates to be entered must have been previously obtained by counting background samples that are physically similar to the unknown samples for long enough to achieve adequate statistical precision.

As the background count rate is dependent upon the channel settings, current counting systems also allow the acquisition of a complete background spectrum (often carried out daily) in order to automatically calculate the required background correction for each energy channel. After the counting channels are determined for any sample, the appropriate background count rate is calculated from this spectrum. This allows any temporal variations or PM drifts to be taken into account.

If the background count rate is a significant fraction of the sample count rate or if background fluctuations occur during the day, then 'blank' background samples should be included in each batch (i.e. before and after the samples to be counted). The counts of these 'blank' samples should then be used to compute the net count rate instead of the use of a preset background correction.

The sample counter's position within a working space and its shielding requirements should be considered as part of system procurement. The proximity to areas where the storage or transport of radioactivity takes place should be considered; this should include waste stores and nuclear medicine injection and therapy rooms. The ambient background levels should be checked as part of the acceptance testing of a new counting system. If a system is to be used for detection of low radiation levels (such as for leak testing) then a stable, preferably low background area is required. In areas with fluctuating background (such as near the patient corridor in a nuclear medicine department), leak-test samples may need to be counted outside working hours to minimise background variability.

When a counting system is to be used for measuring high-energy radionuclides, such as for sample counting of PET tracers, crosstalk between detectors should also be taken into account. Modern multi-detector counters, such as those outlined in section 3.3, are capable of automatically correcting for crosstalk between their detectors. An additional source of background counts is from the racks of samples queuing on the sample counter. As it is difficult to correct for such a transient source of background, it is important to account for the background from these samples when defining the desirable shielding requirements of each detector during procurement. Additionally, one should avoid queuing high-activity samples when counting low-activity samples. Further information on leak tests and on sample counting of high-energy radionuclides is provided in section 10.5.

9.4 Low count rate rejection

If a counter has been set to count a number of samples to a given statistical precision, it may be the case that low-activity samples could take an impractically long time to generate the required counts. Often, such samples are not important anyway (for example, background samples between the peaks of a chromatogram). To prevent the counter from wasting time on such samples, counters often have a facility for the user to enter a count rate below which the sample is to be rejected. One entry per channel should be available on multiple channel counters. The count rate for each sample is checked after a specified time and if it is below the preset rates in all channels, the sample is rejected. This facility should not be used on certain kinds of sample, including background samples, or samples with potentially very low levels of radioactivity, such as leak-test samples. In these cases, it may be preferable to set up a protocol that terminates counting after a specified counting time, instead of terminating after a required number of counts/statistical precision is reached.

9.5 Decay correction

If the time taken to count all the samples is significant compared with the half-life of the radionuclide being assayed, decay correction should be performed. This will correct the count obtained at the sample count time, t_S, to a particular reference time, t_R, through multiplication by a correction factor equal to $e^{0.693\left(\frac{t_S-t_R}{T_{0.5}}\right)}$, where $T_{0.5}$ is the physical half-life of the radionuclide. The uncorrected count should always be recorded in case errors are present in the system or reference date and time or in the assumed half-life; this allows a manual check of the decay correction to be performed. It is also essential to use the uncorrected count in calculations related to statistical counting errors. Additionally, when 'blank' samples are counted within a batch of samples for background correction purposes, the uncorrected counts should be used for the 'blank' samples, i.e. these should not be decay corrected.

Current counters have in-built reference tables of half-lives for different radionuclides. The decay correction capabilities of each counter should be carefully assessed as part of system commissioning, as outlined in chapter 4.

9.6 Efficiency correction for gamma counting

Efficiency correction relates the count rate obtained by the counter to the actual number of disintegrations per second occurring in the sample, i.e. its activity. Factors affecting counting efficiency are discussed in section 1.3.5. An efficiency correction factor or sensitivity in cps/Bq can be derived for any x-ray- or gamma-emitting radionuclide by counting a sample of known activity. In some systems, efficiency correction factors are built in by the manufacturer, and these should be validated during commissioning. The sensitivity of a well-maintained sample counter that is in a stable environment and subject to regular QC checks should be constant for a given radionuclide and sample geometry. Please see chapter 4 for more information on efficiency and constancy checks.

However, it is rare for sample counters to be used for the measurement of sample activity. It is standard and recommended practice within clinical tests to measure the count rates of patient samples in relation to a counting standard, which is itself directly related to the quantity of radiotracer administered to the patient or otherwise used in the test. The relative activity of the patients' samples often differs from that of the standard. If the levels of radioactivity of either the sample or the standard are high enough to cause dead time, the sample may be left to decay to minimise the impact of dead-time effects. Additionally, corrections for dead-time effects may be applied, as outlined in chapter 4.

9.7 Multiple radionuclide counting

9.7.1 Simple dual radionuclide studies

In the simplest case of dual radionuclide counting, in which the counts from the lower-energy nuclide in the higher-energy nuclide channel are negligible, correction for crosstalk from the high-energy radionuclide into the low-energy channel is achieved by counting a high-energy standard in both windows. After background subtraction, the counts in the low-energy window are expressed as a fraction of those in the high-energy window. When counting an unknown sample, the same fraction of the observed high-energy count rate is subtracted from the low-energy count rate to give the net contribution from the low-energy nuclide.

Since crosstalk is usually a result of Compton scattering, it is dependent on sample geometry and density, and so these factors should be kept the same for all standards and samples. Additionally, the crosstalk fraction would have to be re-measured for any change in window settings.

9.7.2 Dual radionuclide studies—general case

Here, a dual radionuclide study general case is presented. Further information for dual radionuclide counting of beta emitters is provided in section 6.11 of the liquid scintillation chapter.

In the general case, if a pure sample of each nuclide is counted in both energy channels and the following count rates are measured:

the count rate of nuclide A in energy window A = n_{AA}
the count rate of nuclide A in energy window B = n_{AB}
the count rate of nuclide B in energy window A = n_{BA}
the count rate of nuclide B in energy window B = n_{BB}
and if:
the count rate of the sample in energy window A = n_{SA}
the count rate of the sample in energy window B = n_{SB}

then the count rates n_A and n_B that would have been obtained from each nuclide separately in any unknown sample can be deduced by solving the simultaneous equations:

$$n_{SA} = n_A + \frac{n_{BA}}{n_{BB}} n_B$$

$$n_{SB} = \frac{n_{AB}}{n_{AA}} n_A + n_B.$$

Reference

2002 The Medical Devices Regulations, UK Statutory Instrument 2002 No. 618. Published by The National Archives on behalf of HM Government. https://www.legislation.gov.uk/uksi/2002/618/contents/made

Chapter 10

Clinical and research applications of sample counters

Peter O'Sullivan, Sofia Michopoulou, Andrew Fenwick, Lucy Pike, Anne-Marie Stapleton and Fergus McKiddie

10.1 Introduction

This chapter provides a collection of practical worked examples outlining clinical and research applications of radioactivity sample counters. These are intended to provide typical counting parameters and highlight technical considerations for a range of applications.

An overview of glomerular filtration estimation is provided in section 10.2, which outlines a typical sample preparation and counting technique for this study, while section 10.3 outlines methods for calculating uncertainties in measurements of glomerular filtration rate. Section 10.4 discusses the derivation of input functions using arterial blood sampling. Section 10.5 describes the use of gamma counters for radiopharmaceutical quality control and provides an example of the measurement of breakthrough in germanium-68/gallium-68 generation. Section 10.6 focuses on radiation protection aspects and recommends instruments and techniques for counting leak-test samples and characterising radioactive contamination. Section 10.7 discusses dual-isotope counting using a gamma counter and section 10.8 outlines sample volume effects in gamma counting. Section 10.9 provides an example of blood sample counting for radionuclide therapy dosimetry, and finally, section 10.10 provides a worked example of using quality control charts.

10.2 Glomerular filtration rate measurements

The following worked example of a typical glomerular filtration rate (GFR) calculation uses the single-sample technique recommended in the BNMS clinical guideline released in 2018 (Burniston 2018). This was a change from the previous

doi:10.1088/978-0-7503-3895-0ch10

guidance, which recommended the multi-sample slope-intercept technique. These common calculations will generally be carried out using standard spreadsheets or software programmes written specifically for the task. The process of creating and validating these should be subject to a suitable quality assessment system, as described in section 9.2. Manual calculations, as illustrated here, are useful for the testing and validation of automated calculation methods.

The single-sample technique has the advantage of requiring fewer blood samples from the patient, which improves the patient experience. Recent studies have also developed robust quality control processes for this technique and demonstrated that it can be as accurate and precise as the multi-sample methods.

The patient should be adequately hydrated at the time of the test, have a light breakfast and, if possible, caffeinated drinks should be avoided from 10 pm the previous evening. High-protein meals should be avoided before and during the test, as a protein load can alter the reproducibility of the result. Any medication which may alter or interfere with renal function should be noted.

The patient attends the department, and after their identification is checked, in accordance with IR(ME)R, their height and weight are measured to allow calculation of an accurate body surface area (BSA). The patient's age and sex should also be noted to allow calculation of the age- and sex-specific expected normal ranges. In this example, the patient was a male 40 years old, 1.65 m tall, and 94.5 kg in weight.

Two syringes were dispensed from the radiopharmacy, both containing the same concentration of ^{99m}Tc-DTPA (diethylenetriamine pentaacetate) (the first is for administration to the patient and the second syringe is used for the creation of a counting standard). The patient and standard syringes were weighed in their full state on a calibrated balance and found to weigh 3.738 and 3.722 g, respectively. The patient was injected with 5.23 MBq from the first syringe, and the injection site and time were noted: 08.51 am, injection into a vein in the right wrist. The standard solution was created and the patient and standard syringes were then weighed in their empty state on the same calibrated balance and found to weigh 3.284 and 3.27 g, respectively.

The patient was then allowed to leave the department and asked to return in sufficient time for a blood sample to be taken 4 h after the injection. If the patient is anticipated to have impaired renal function, additional samples can be taken at later timepoints or the sampling can be delayed. In this case there were no clinical indications of any impairment to renal function, so sampling was carried out using the standard timing. Recommended timings based on the expected GFR can be found in the BNMS guideline, but the single-sample calculation method described in the guideline can be used for samples taken at 2, 3, 4, or 6 h.

A blood sample was taken from the opposite arm to that used for the injection, in this case the left arm, into a heparinised blood tube. The time of the sample was noted exactly, which was 12.52. The sample tube was placed in a centrifuge and spun at 1000 g for 10 min to separate the packed red blood cells from the plasma.

Two 1 mL samples of plasma were taken from the spun blood tube and placed in sample tubes for the gamma counter. Two sample tubes were filled to 1 mL with water for backgrounds. Four 1 mL aliquots of the standard solution were taken and placed in separate sample tubes. All sample tubes were placed in the appropriate counting rack and placed on the gamma counter. The time was noted when the first sample started to count to allow for decay correction in the processing. In this case the counting start time was 14.31. Each sample was counted for 5 min. The gamma counter was set to decay correct all sample results relative to the time at which the counting started for the first sample.

The first task was to calculate the apparent volume of distribution v_{app} from the ratio of the sample and standard counts; this reflects the dilution which has occurred. The equation used was

$$v_{app} = \frac{\text{corrected standard cpm} \times \text{dose to standard ratio} \times \text{standard volume (mL)}}{\text{corrected sample cpm}}.$$

The ratio of the injected volumes for the patient and standard, i.e. the dose-to-standard ratio, was calculated using

$$\text{Ratio} = \frac{3.738{-}3.284}{3.722{-}3.27} = 1.0044.$$

The average decay and background-corrected counts in cpm mL^{-1} for the patient sample and standard were found to be as follows:

Sample type	Average result
Standard	244 489.65
Patient sample	1682.75

The apparent volume of distribution was thus

$$v_{app} = \frac{244489.65 \times 1.0044 \times 1000}{1682.75} = 145931\text{mL}.$$

This was then converted into a result in litres and normalised to the standard body surface of 1.73 m^2. This first required the patient's BSA to be calculated. Several different formulae are available for this, but the guidelines recommend Haycock's method, which states that

$$\text{BSA}(m^2) = 0.024265 \times \text{weight(kg)}^{0.5378} \times \text{height(cm)}^{0.3964}.$$

Inserting the measurements taken earlier for this patient gave:

$$\text{BSA}(m^2) = 0.024265 \times 94.5^{0.5378} \times 165^{0.3964} = 2.12 \quad m^2.$$

The normalised v_{app_norm} was then calculated as follows:

$$v_{app\_norm} = v_{app} \times \frac{1.73}{1000 \times \text{BSA}} = 119.09 \frac{\text{L}}{1.73} m^2.$$

The equation given in the guidelines for the calculation of the GFR is:

$$\text{GFR} = \frac{1}{t} \times \big((-11297 - (4883 \times \text{BSA}) - (41.9 \times t)) + (5862 + (1282 \times \text{BSA}) + (15.5 \times t) \times \ln v_{app\_norm})\big),$$

where t is the time between the injection and the sample, which in this case is 241 min.

Substituting in the calculated values gives:

$$\text{GFR} = \frac{1}{241} \times ((-11297 - (4883 \times 2.12) - (41.9 \times 241))$$
$$+ (5862 + (1282 \times 2.12) + (15.5 \times 241) \times \ln 119.09)) = 112.5 \quad \text{mL}/\frac{\text{min}}{1.73\text{m}^2}.$$

It should be noted that this calculated value is normalised for the BSA. If required, this can then be converted back to the patient's BSA to produce the final absolute GFR measurement. In this case, this gives

$$\text{GFR}_{\text{abs}} = \text{GFR} \times \frac{\text{BSA}}{1.73} = 112.5 \times \frac{2.12}{1.73} = 137.9\text{mL/ min}.$$

There are age-related expected normal values which can be calculated and displayed alongside the absolute patient result to guide clinicians, as discussed in the BNMS guidelines. The exact combination of results provided to the referring clinicians is best discussed with them by each department and the output tailored to their requirements. Renal physicians working in adult services often prefer the absolute value, as do pharmacists for chemotherapy dosage calculation, while paediatric renal physicians often prefer the BSA-normalised value, as this accounts for growth during childhood.

10.3 Calculation of the uncertainties in the measurement of glomerular filtration rate in patients

The glomerular filtration rate (GFR) is a clinical measurement of the kidneys commonly assessed using radionuclides. The methodology and calculation is described in detail in the BNMS clinical guidelines (Burniston 2018). The most recent version of these clinical guidelines recommends the methodology characterised by the use of a single plasma sample. In this section we will attempt to assess the uncertainties associated with this calculation.

This example will use the same data and equations as those described in section 9.2. Please refer to that section for a fuller description of the calculation.

The GFR is calculated using the following equations:

$$\text{GFR}\left[\frac{\text{mL}}{\text{min}}/1.73\text{m}^2\right]$$
$$= \left(\frac{1}{t[\text{min}]}\right) \times \left\{(-11297 + (4883 \times \text{BSA}[\text{m}^2]) + 41.9t[\text{min}])\right.$$
$$\left. + [5862 + (1282 \times \text{BSA}[\text{m}^2]) + 15.5t[\text{min}]]\text{Ln}\left(\text{V}_{\text{app\_norm}}\left[\frac{1}{1.73\text{m}^2}\right]\right)\right\}$$

$$\text{GFR}_{\text{abs}} = \text{GFR} \times \left(\frac{\text{BSA}}{1.73}\right) \quad \text{V}_{\text{app\_norm}}\left[\frac{l}{1.73\text{m}^2}\right] = \frac{1.73[\text{m}^2]}{1000\text{BSA}[\text{m}^2]}$$

$$V_{\text{app}}[\text{mL}] = \frac{\text{corrected standard cpm}\left[\frac{\text{cpm}}{\text{mL}}\right] \times \text{dose to standard ratio} \times \text{standard volume[mL]}}{\text{corrected sample cpm}\left[\frac{\text{cpm}}{\text{mL}}\right]}$$

$$\text{BSA}[\text{m}^2] = 0.024265 \times \text{Weight[kg]}^{0.5378} \times \text{Height[cm]}^{0.3964},$$

where:

V_{app} is the apparent volume of distribution
$V_{\text{app\_norm}}$ is the normalised apparent volume of distribution
BSA is the body surface area
cpm is the counts per minute
Bgd is the background
Weight standard injection, W_s ($W_s = W_{\text{sfull}} - W_{\text{sempty}}$)
Weight patient injection, W_p ($W_p = W_{\text{pfull}} - W_{\text{pempty}}$)
Sample time, t ($t = t_s - t_i$)
GFR is the BSA-normalised GFR in units of mL $\text{min}^{-1}/1.73\ \text{m}^2$
GFR_{abs} is the non-BSA-normalised GFR in units of mL min^{-1}
σ is the standard deviation
$\sigma_F(\%)$ is the fractional standard deviation

The raw data is presented in table 10.1 and a breakdown of the components used in the uncertainty calculation is presented in table 10.2.

$$^{*}\sigma(V_{\text{app}}) = (V_{\text{app}}) \cdot \sqrt{\left(\frac{\sigma(C_s)}{C_s}\right)^2 + \left(\frac{\sigma(C_p)}{C_p}\right)^2 + \left(\frac{\sigma(R)}{R}\right)^2 + \left(\frac{\sigma(V_s)}{V_s}\right)^2}$$

$$^{**}\text{BSA} = 0.024265\text{Wt}^{0.5378} \times \text{Ht}^{0.3964};$$

$$\text{let } a = 0.024265\text{Wt}^{0.5378} \text{ and } b = \text{Ht}^{0.3964}$$

$$\text{then,} \quad \sigma(a) = 0.5378(\sigma(\text{Wt})/\text{Wt}) \quad \text{and} \quad \sigma(b) = 0.3964(\sigma(\text{Ht})/\text{Ht})$$

$$\text{and,} \quad \sigma(\text{BSA}) = \text{BSA} \cdot \sqrt{((\sigma(a)/a))^2 + ((\sigma(b)/b))^2}$$

$$^{***}\sigma(V_{\text{app\_norm}}) = (V_{\text{app\_norm}}) \cdot \sqrt{\left(\frac{\sigma(\text{BSA})}{\text{BSA}}\right)^2 + \left(\frac{\sigma(V_{\text{app}})}{V_{\text{app}}}\right)^2 + \left(\frac{\sigma(V_s)}{V_s}\right)^2}$$

****For more complex equations, such as those used to calculate the GFR, substitution simplifies the task of propagating uncertainties, see table 10.3.

$$\text{GFR} = \frac{L}{t} = \left(\frac{1}{t}\right) \cdot (G + K) = \left(\frac{1}{t}\right) \cdot (G + H \cdot J) = \left(\frac{1}{t}\right) \cdot \left(G + H \cdot Ln\left(V_{\text{app\_norm}}\right)\right),$$

$$\text{where } G = a_1 + (a_2 \cdot \text{BSA}) + a_3 \cdot t \text{ and } H = b_1 + (b_2 \cdot \text{BSA}) + b_3 \cdot t.$$

Table 10.1. The raw data required for the GFR calculation.

Values			Uncertainty in values		
Quantity	Value	Unit	Symbol	σ	$\sigma_F(\%)$
Height, Ht	165	cm	$\sigma(\text{Height})$	1	0.6
Weight, Wt	94.5	kg	$\sigma(\text{Weight})$	0.5	0.5
Weight of full standard syringe, W_{sfull}	3.722	g	$\sigma(W_{\text{sfull}})$	0.005	0.13
Weight of empty standard syringe, W_{sempty}	3.270	g	$\sigma(W_{\text{sempty}})$	0.005	0.15
Weight of full patient syringe, W_{pfull}	3.738	g	$\sigma(W_{\text{pfull}})$	0.005	0.13
Weight of empty patient syringe, W_{pempty}	3.284	g	$\sigma(W_{\text{pempty}})$	0.005	0.15
Volume of standard, V_s	1000	mL	$\sigma(V_s)$	1	0.1
Time of injection, t_i	10:00		$\sigma(t_i)$	1 min	
Time of sample, t_s	14:01		$\sigma(t_s)$	1 min	
Standard + bgd cpm (C_{s+b})	244 525	cpm	$\sigma(C_{s+b})$	$\sqrt{\left(\frac{C_{s+b}}{t_{\text{sct}}}\right)} = 156.4$	0.06
Patient sample + bgd cpm (C_{p+b})	1718	cpm	$\sigma(C_{p+b})$	$\sqrt{\left(\frac{C_{p+b}}{t_{\text{sct}}}\right)} = 13.1$	0.76
bgd cpm (C_b)	35.6	cpm	$\sigma(C_b)$	$\sqrt{\left(\frac{C_b}{t_{\text{sct}}}\right)} = 1.89$	5.30
Sample counting time, t_{sct}	10	min			

Table 10.2. The calculated uncertainties in each of the calculation components.

Values			Uncertainty in values			
Quantity	Value	Unit	Symbol	Calculation	σ	$\sigma_F(\%)$
Weight of standard injection, W_s	0.452	g	$\sigma(W_s)$	$\sqrt{\sigma(W_{sfull})^2 + \sigma(W_{sempty})^2}$	0.0071	1.56
Weight of patient injection, W_p	0.454	g	$\sigma(W_p)$	$\sqrt{\sigma(W_{pfull})^2 + \sigma(W_{pempty})^2}$	0.0071	1.56
Sample time, t	241	min	$\sigma(t)$	$\sqrt{\sigma(t_i)^2 + \sigma(t_s)^2}$	1.41	0.59
Standard—bgd counts, C_s	244 490	cpm	$\sigma(C_s)$	$\sqrt{\sigma(C_{s+b})^2 + \sigma(C_b)^2}$	156.4	0.06
Patient—bgd counts, C_p	1683	cpm	$\sigma(C_p)$	$\sqrt{\sigma(C_{p+b})^2 + \sigma(C_b)^2}$	13.24	0.79
Ratio, R (= W_p/W_s)	1.004 42		$\sigma(R)$	$\left(\frac{W_p}{W_s}\right)\cdot\sqrt{\left(\frac{\sigma(W_p)}{W_p}\right)^2 + \left(\frac{\sigma(W_s)}{W_s}\right)^2}$	0.02	2.21
V_{app}	145 934	mL	$\sigma(V_{app})$	*	34 24.5	2.35
BSA	2.120	m^2	σ(BSA)	**	0.02	1.02
V_{app_norm}	119.1	l/1.73 m^2	$\sigma(V_{app\_norm})$	***	3.05	2.56
GFR	112.5	mL min^{-1}/1.73 m^2	σ(GFR)	****	1.47	1.30
GFR_{abs}	137.9	mL min^{-1}	$\sigma(GFR_{abs})$	$(GFR_{abs})\cdot\sqrt{\left(\frac{\sigma(GFR)}{GFR}\right)^2 + \left(\frac{\sigma(BSA)}{BSA}\right)^2}$	2.28	1.65

Table 10.3. Calculation of the uncertainties in the GFR using substitution.

Values		Uncertainty in values		
Quantity	Value	Symbol	Calculation	σ
G	−31 748	σ(G)	$\sqrt{\sigma(\text{BSA})^2 + \sigma(t)^2}$	1.41
H	12 316	σ(H)	$\sqrt{\sigma(\text{BSA})^2 + \sigma(t)^2}$	1.41
J	4.7798	σ(J)	$\sigma\left(V_{\text{app norm}}\right)/V_{\text{app norm}}$	0.0256
K	58 866	σ(K)	$(K)\cdot\sqrt{\left(\frac{\sigma(H)}{H}\right)^2 + \left(\frac{\sigma(J)}{J}\right)^2}$	315.3
L	27 118	σ(L)	$\sqrt{\sigma(G)^2 + \sigma(K)^2}$	315.3
GFR	112.5	σ(GFR)	$(\text{GFR})\cdot\sqrt{\left(\frac{\sigma(t)}{t}\right)^2 + \left(\frac{\sigma(L)}{L}\right)^2}$	1.47

This assessment relates to the uncertainties of the defined raw data and can be a useful tool in understanding the potential uncertainties in the controllable factors involved in a procedure of this kind. In order to calculate the total uncertainty, this assessment would have to be combined with the uncertainty related to the empirical modelling of the single-sample data to the initial multi-sample methods, and the underlying clinical variability due to number of different physiological systems.

It is recommended that an assessment of the uncertainties of any new procedure is undertaken as part of the commissioning process. It is especially important that the impact of the uncertainties in the controllable factors is understood and managed as part of the clinical procedure.

10.4 Quantitation in PET using arterial-blood-derived input functions

Most clinical studies in Nuclear Medicine and PET use relative quantification, in which the count rate in the patient samples or images is measured at a particular timepoint and compared to a reference. PET can be acquired in dynamic mode, in which the functional data is binned as a function of time so that the kinetics of the tracer can be measured in the tissues or organs of interest. Using certain radiotracers, this allows the *in vivo* measurement of a number of physiological processes, such as glucose metabolism, cerebral blood flow, and receptor binding.

Acquired PET images are made up of superimposed information from the radiotracer as it travels in the blood and enters different states within the physiological system. To isolate the desired component of the PET signal, compartmental modelling is used to describe the system as a function of time (Morris *et al* 2004). To mathematically model the system in this way, a measured input function that describes the delivery of the parent radiotracer into the system is essential. By comparing the output of the model to the measured input, the kinetic parameters of the system can then be estimated. The review by Morris *et al* (2004) provides a useful overview of some of the compartmental models used in PET and sources for further reading, and the reader is directed to the Turku PET Centre website, which includes an Introduction to Modelling section written by Vesa Oikonen (2011).

There are several ways to measure the input function, but most research applications of PET sample the arterial blood over the course of the PET study (Cunningham *et al* 2004) and this is considered the gold standard. The fraction of parent tracer in arterial blood is derived from an assay of the activity in the plasma. This example outlines the steps required to obtain and process arterial blood in order to derive the input function. The PMOD Application Note (Turku PET Centre 2019) provides detailed protocols for obtaining blood data for PET quantitation in animal and human applications.

10.4.1 Method

As timing is critical to the accuracy of the quantification, a stopwatch or reference clock should be used for all timings. In an ideal setup, all equipment (PET scanner, gamma counter, automatic blood sample counter) and clocks in the scanning department should be connected to a NTP (network time protocol) server so that they are synchronised. If this is not available, the clocks in all the equipment can either be synchronised prior to the study, or a stopwatch (and back up) used to record all timings. In this case, a record of the times shown by the equipment relative to the stopwatch should be made prior to starting the study, so that these can be used to correct the timings of all subsequent measurements relative to the injection time. The gamma counter used to count the components from the manual blood samples should be cross-calibrated to the PET scanner (so that both yield kBq mL^{-1}).

The patient is positioned in the PET scanner with an arterial line *in situ,* usually in the radial artery. A CT for attenuation correction is acquired over the region of interest and the bed moved ready to start the PET scan. The automatic blood sampling system is started, and the arterial blood is continuously pumped through the radiation detectors. The dynamic PET acquisition is started. The patient is then injected with the radiotracer, which is usually performed as a rapid intravenous bolus injection, and the time recorded.

The arterial blood is continuously sampled for the first few minutes to capture the initial peak. After this, manual blood samples are drawn from the arterial line using a three-way tap at specific timepoints and the actual time recorded. The initial timepoints for the manual samples should overlap with the continuous sampling, as they are used to calibrate the output from the continuous arterial sampling, but manual samples should not be taken too early, so as to avoid disrupting the measurement of the initial peak.

An aliquot of arterial whole blood from the manual samples is spun in a centrifuge to separate the plasma. Aliquots of plasma and whole blood are then pipetted into separate vials and counted in the gamma counter. If present, metabolites are separated from the plasma using chromatography or cartridge techniques and the components counted in the gamma counter.

10.4.2 Data processing

To generate the time–activity curve for the tissue of interest (figure 10.1), a region of interest (ROI) is drawn on the area in the reconstructed PET images. Using summed frames, or later time frames, can help to visualise the tissue of interest for segmenting and the ROI can be copied across all frames. The activity concentration in the tissue can either be taken as the mean over the ROI, or voxel-wise analysis can be performed. The activity concentration should be decay corrected to the time of injection, unless this is automatically performed by the scanner.

The automatic blood sampling system measures the activity concentration in the whole blood with a high temporal resolution (typically 1 s) to capture the initial bolus of radiotracer (figure 10.2). This data is decay corrected and adjusted to the PET injection time. The counts per second (CPS) from the manual samples are corrected for background, dead time, and crosstalk; they are decay corrected to the injection time, and the cross-calibration factor is applied to convert the CPS to an activity concentration (kBq mL^{-1}). The activity concentration measured in the whole blood from the manual samples is used to calibrate the curve from the automatic blood sampling system, and mathematical models are used to interpolate between the discrete timepoints.

To determine the tracer in the plasma only and not that bound to red blood cells and large proteins, a plasma correction needs to be applied to the arterial whole-blood data. The counts from the manual samples are used to determine the plasma-to-whole-blood ratio at each timepoint (figure 10.3).

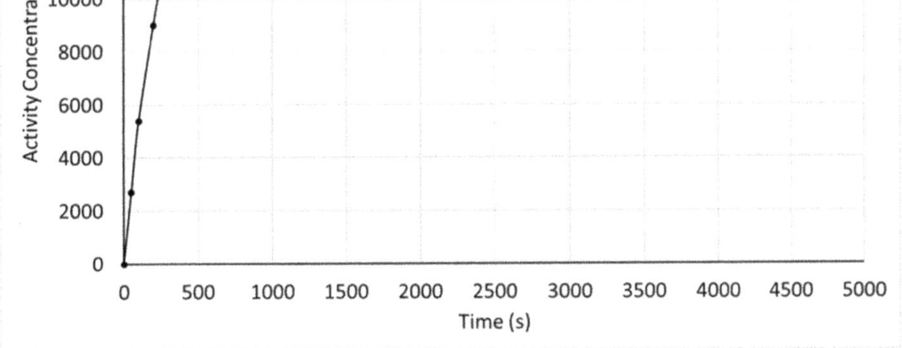

Figure 10.1. Simulated time–activity curve showing the mean tracer activity concentration measured in the tissue of interest over time from PET images.

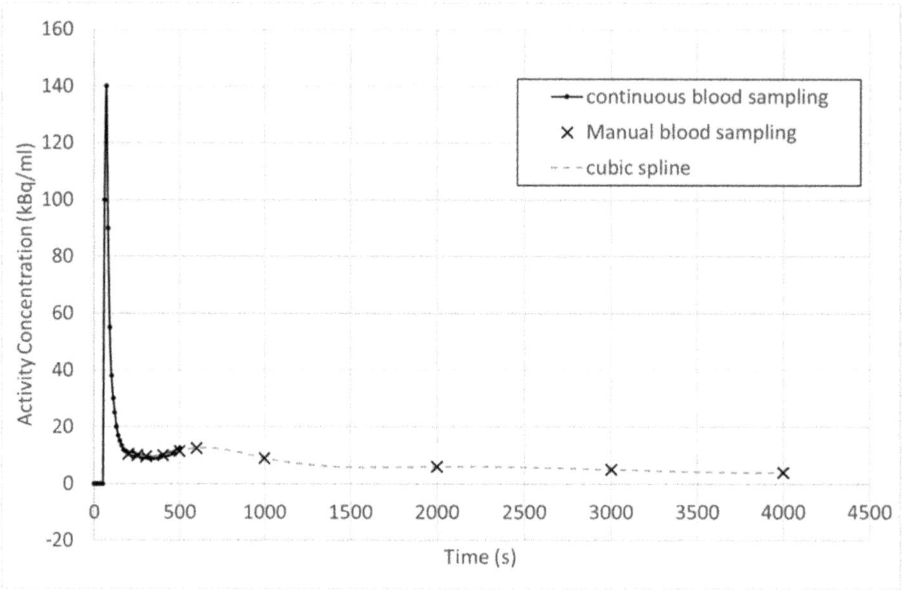

Figure 10.2. Example plot of tracer activity concentration measured in arterial blood using continuous sampling (solid line) and manual samples (crosses).

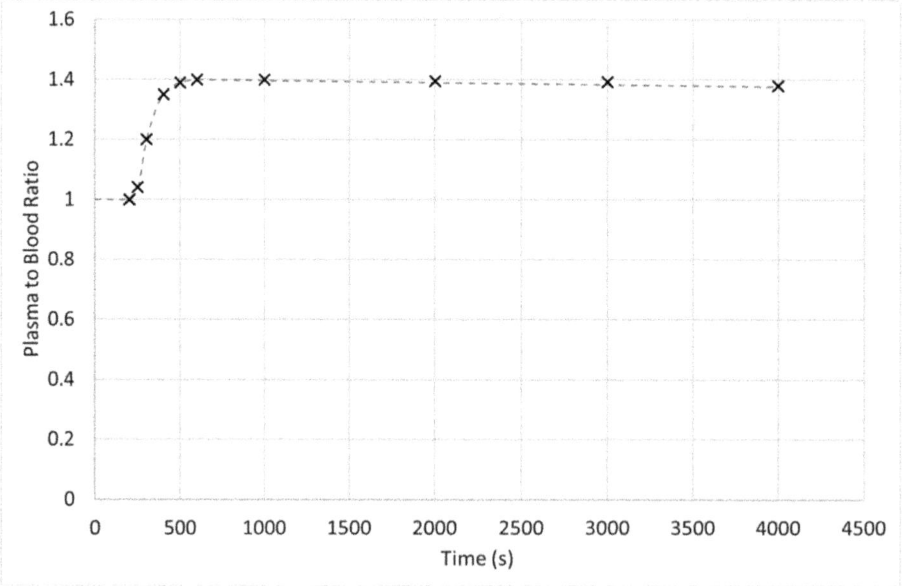

Figure 10.3. Example plot of plasma-to-blood ratio determined from an assay of manual blood samples.

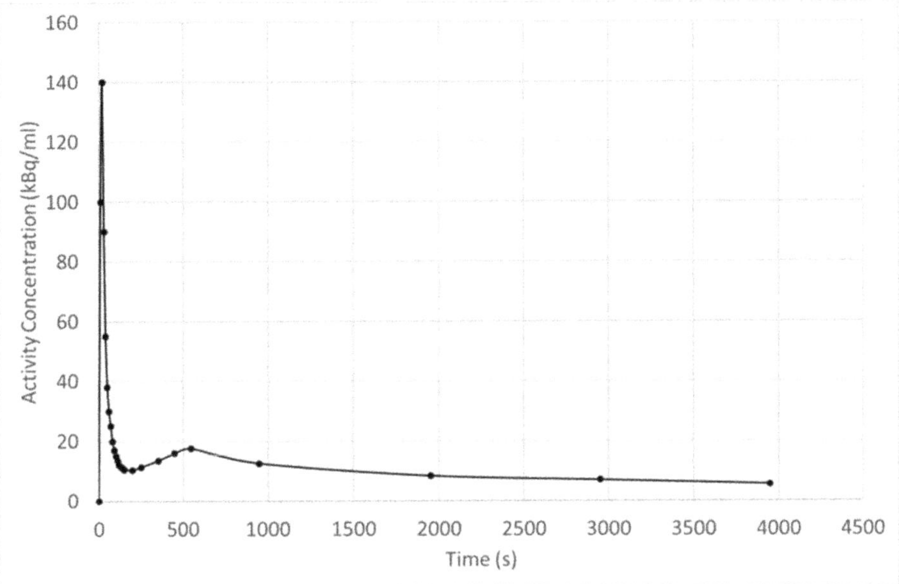

Figure 10.4. Plot of total plasma activity concentration.

The whole-blood curve is multiplied by the plasma-to-whole-blood ratio to determine the plasma activity concentration curve (figure 10.4).

Some radiotracers are metabolised in the body, and this will contribute to the counts in the plasma. This may be observed as a small peak in the total plasma curve, just after the initial peak (figure 10.4). To account for metabolites, the plasma from the manual blood samples is measured using high-performance liquid chromatography (or, where validated, using a cartridge-based method) to separate the components from the parent and the metabolites. To determine the fraction that is not metabolised (the parent fraction) at each timepoint, the area of the parent peak is divided by the total area for all the metabolite peaks. The rate and mechanism of metabolism of the parent is tracer dependent, and not all tracers are metabolised, e.g. fluorodeoxyglucose (FDG). An example of what a parent fraction curve may look like is shown in figure 10.5.

The total plasma curve is multiplied by the parent fraction in the plasma curve to give the final parent plasma input function (figure 10.6). If the radiotracer is not metabolised, as is the case, for example, for FDG, this step is not required.

The TAC from the PET images and the parent plasma input function derived from the arterial sampling are then used as inputs into the kinetic model and the physiological parameters are estimated.

There is a delay between the time that the tracer enters the tissue of interest and the time of measurement in the detectors of the automatic blood sampling system. This is known as dispersion, and it varies depending on the tracer. If significant, dispersion needs to be corrected for.

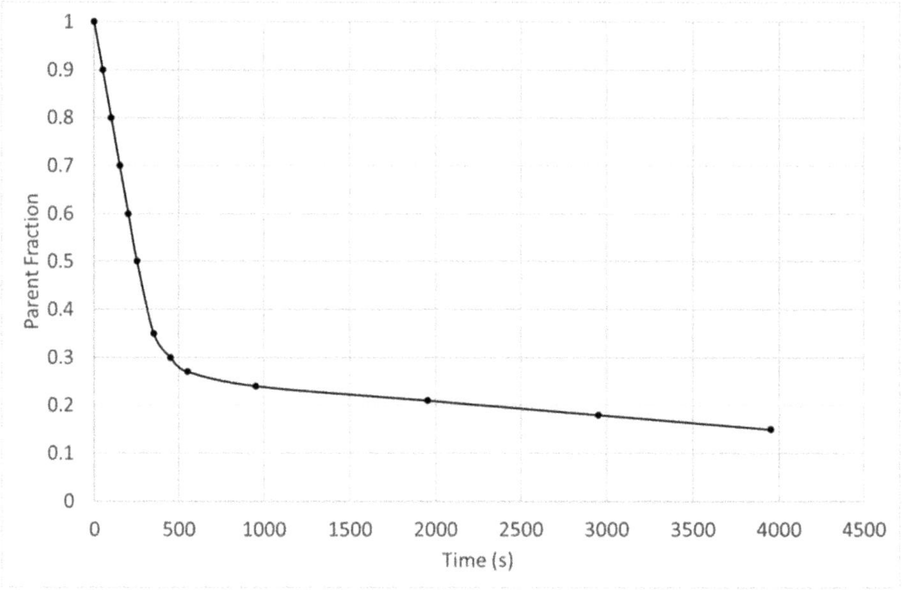

Figure 10.5. Plot of a parent fraction.

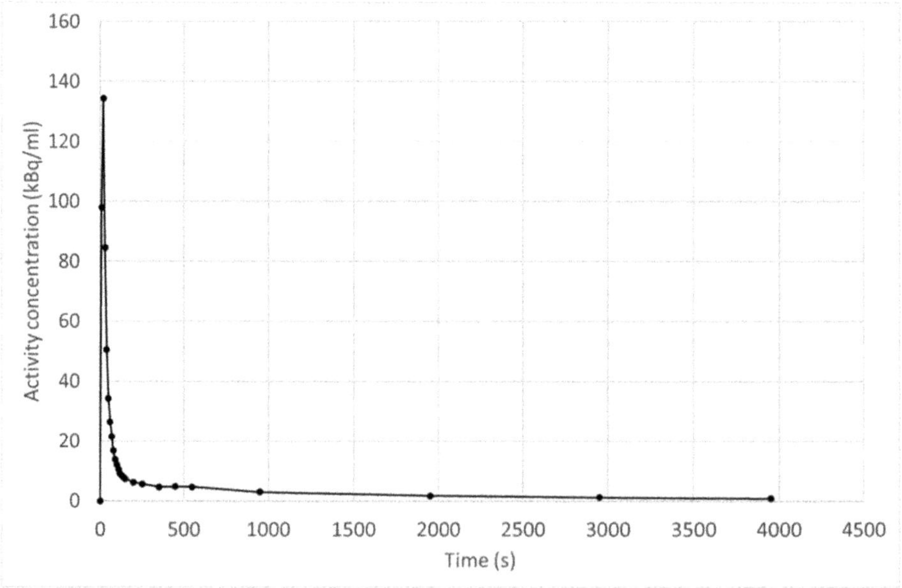

Figure 10.6. Simulated parent plasma input function.

10.5 Measurement of ^{68}Ge breakthrough from a Ge/^{68}Ga generator

Ge/^{68}Ga generators are routinely used to produce ^{68}Ga for PET imaging. The parent isotope, germanium-68, has a half-life of 271 days, while the half-life of the daughter isotope, gallium-68, is 68 min. Ge/^{68}Ga generators have a glass column where the parent radionuclide is fixed (adsorbed) on the sorbent, so that the daughter radionuclide can be eluted by passing hydrochloric acid solution through the column. During elution, a small quantity of ^{68}Ge breaks through to the eluate. Due to the long half-life of ^{68}Ge, it is important to ensure that the breakthrough is as small as possible in order to reduce the radiation dose given to patients injected with ^{68}Ga solution. The European Pharmacopoeia specifies that ^{68}Ge breakthrough should be less than 0.001% of the eluted activity (Vis *et al* 2015).

Breakthrough can be measured by assaying a sample from the eluate using a gamma counter. During counting the energy window should be centred at 511 keV. Two measurements should be taken, one at ~15 h, and one at ~60 h after generator elution. The 15 h timepoint is used to establish a measurement for the original eluted ^{68}Ga, including the breakthrough ^{68}Ge. At the 60 h' timepoint, the original eluted ^{68}Ga has decayed and the resulting measurement corresponds to the breakthrough ^{68}Ge, which has reached equilibrium with the ^{68}Ga. A background measurement should be taken before and after each sample measurement. As the breakthrough ratio is very low, it is recommended to use a long sample acquisition time at 60 h. The measurements at 15 h and 60 h are decay corrected back to the elution time to quantify the ratio of ^{68}Ga activity and ^{68}Ge breakthrough (Green *et al* 2016). An example calculation is outlined here.

Example Breakthrough Counting Protocol:
Radionuclide: ^{68}Ge
Decay correction: off
Background correction: on.
Sample counting durations: 5 min at 15 h, 60 min at 60 h
Calculation based on 0.1 mL sample taken directly from the eluate (~10 MBq ^{68}Ga)

Sample	Count duration (sec)	BKG corrected total counts	CPM
@15 h	300	97 722	19 544
@60 h	3600	52 426	874

The ^{68}Ga derived counts at 15 h can be calculated by subtracting the decay-corrected ^{68}Ge component.

^{68}Ga @ 15 h = 19 544–874 * $e^{\ln(2) * 45/24/271}$ = 18 666 CPM.

Finally, the individual ^{68}Ga and ^{68}Ge activities at 0 h can be calculated by decay correction of the derived ^{68}Ga counts at 15 h and the measured ^{68}Ge counts at 60 h:

^{68}Ga @ elution = 18 666 * $e^{\ln(2) * 15 * 60/68}$ = 179 997 761 CPM,

^{68}Ge @ elution = 874 * $e^{\ln(2) * 60/24/271}$ = 880 CPM,

Germanium breakthrough = 880/179 997 761 = 0.000 49%.

An alternative approach to breakthrough assay involves the measurement of a sample against a standard ^{68}Ge source (such as a National Institute of Standards and Technology (NIST) traceable test source). The ^{68}Ge standard source allows the detection efficiency of a gamma counter to be determined (which is typically ~30% for a standard-sized NaI(T) crystal) (Lodge *et al* 2015). The sample can then be measured once at 60 h after elution and the germanium breakthrough activity calculated by applying a correction factor for detection efficiency. Finally, the measured ^{68}Ge activity should be expressed as a percentage of the ^{68}Ga activity measured by a radionuclide calibration at the time of elution (Amor-Coarasa *et al* 2016).

10.6 Leak-test counting using a gamma counter

Under regulation 28(3) of the Ionising Radiations Regulations 2017, leak testing must be performed on sealed sources at least every two years, or more frequently if this is identified as a recommendation in the risk assessment.

The choice of an appropriate leak-testing methodology will depend on the type of sealed source and the encapsulation of the source; guidance can be found in ISO 9978: Radiation protection—Sealed radioactive sources—Leakage test methods. This section will concentrate on wipe leak-test methods.

10.6.1 Wipe-test methodology

Before commencing leak testing, the operator must ensure that the correct technique and equipment are used and that the potential exposure that could be caused by leak testing the source has been calculated and justified. If practicable, the sealed source should be cleaned prior to testing.

The wipe should be made of highly absorbent material, and as long as doing so will not damage the encapsulation of the source, it should be moistened with water or ethanol. All the external surfaces of the sealed source should be thoroughly wiped. It may be necessary to use multiple swabs on larger sources.

Typically, a leak test is assessed in two stages. Both stages require the use of a sample counter with a threshold of detectability of the order of 10–1 Bq. Most radionuclide sample counters are easily capable of reaching these thresholds for typical gamma-emitting radionuclides.

The samples are counted with an open window (15–2000 keV); this will ensure that any detectable radioactivity will be included in the assessment. The samples must be counted alongside a sufficient number of background samples. Ideally, the background samples should be measured in between the leak-test samples.

As was discussed in chapter 5, the standard error of the mean of any number of single counts is essentially the same as the standard error of a single count of equal total time. However, counting multiple samples gives an indication of the stability of the counter and whether the background is changing significantly during the exercise. A simple way of assessing this is to count ten background samples and see whether 6–7 of the results fall within ±1 square root of the mean and whether these samples are distributed throughout the exercise.

The counting time for the leak-test samples and the background samples should be the same (as the expected counts in both sets of samples are of the same order) and should be evaluated to achieve a specified percentage standard error. For example, to achieve a percentage standard error of 1%, the samples would have to be counted for a sufficient time to achieve at least 10 000 counts.

The leak-test samples' results should be examined in relation to the mean background counts. Sample counts within three standard deviations of the mean background count can be considered to be leaktight. If the sample counts are greater than this, then this requires further investigation.

In order to assess samples with measured counts greater than these levels, a criterion is required that sets an activity threshold, depending on the leak-testing method used, for a leaktight source. The approval criterion used in ISO 9978 is a detected activity of 0.2 kBq present on both a dry and wet wipe, below which, the source can be considered to be leaktight. It is still important to determine the origin of detected activity below these thresholds, especially if it is arising from source leakage. This could involve repeating the leak testing (subject to satisfactory radiation protection assessment) and monitoring whether the level of detected activity increases.

If counts greater than three standard deviations from the mean background count are measured, it is important to review the full spectrum from that sample to see whether a particular photopeak and hence a specific radionuclide can be identified. The efficiency of the sample counter is radionuclide dependent, as the efficiency varies with energy and the abundance of a particular radionuclide emission.

For convenience, the activity estimate can be made using the same open window (15–2000 keV) count; this is particularly the case if a manufacturer's estimate of the radionuclide efficiency is made using an open window.

In order to convert the measured counts on the swab to an activity estimate, a calibration factor is required. Ideally, this can be measured using a known activity of the same radionuclide, and with an activity low enough that dead-time effects are either negligible or are suitably modelled and corrected in the software. If this is not possible, the sample counter manufacturer will usually state efficiencies for a range of radionuclides.

If it is suspected that a leak wipe contains multiple radionuclides, seek advice from the Radiation Protection Advisor (RPA) and/or Health Physics.

10.6.2 Worked example

Twelve leak-test swabs were counted in a sample counter interspersed with background samples. The samples were counted with an open window and for 3600 s each.

Background samples		Samples		
ID	Total counts	ID	Total counts	Result
bk1	9946	A	10 166	Pass
bk2	10 619	B	10 134	Pass
bk3	10 027	C	10 201	Pass
bk4	10 157	D	10 124	Pass
bk5	9888	E	9826	Pass
bk6	10 418	F	10 123	Pass
bk7	10 169	G	10 027	Pass
bk8	10 676	H	10 157	Pass
bk9	10 126	I	9888	Pass
bk10	10 455	J	10 494	Pass
		K	11 250	Fail
Average	**10 248**	L	12 500	Fail
# of BG	10			
SD	301			
3SD	902			
Mean + 3SD	11 150			
No. within +/− $\sqrt{N}$	6			

All of the samples except K and L have measured counts that are within three standard deviations from the mean background count, and can therefore be regarded as leaktight.

Samples K and L were taken from ^{137}Cs and ^{57}Co sources, respectively, and are further assessed by comparing the measured counts against the manufacturer's stated efficiency values. Alternatively, if a source of known activity of either radionuclide (of appropriate activity and size for the sample counter) were available, then this could be used to obtain a calibration factor.

The manufacturer states efficiencies of 44% and 85% for ^{137}Cs and ^{57}Co, respectively. These can be used to convert the total counts of the samples to activity using the following equation:

$$\text{Activity (Bq)} = \frac{(\text{Sample counts} - \text{background}) \times (100/\text{efficiency}(\%)\ \ )}{\text{Counting time(s)}}.$$

Samples				
ID	Total counts—bgd	Source	Efficiency, %	Activity estimate, Bq
K	1002	^{137}Cs	44	0.6
L	2252	^{57}Co	85	4.1

The activity estimates for both samples are well below the 200 Bq limit and therefore both sources can be considered to be leaktight.

10.7 Dual radionuclide counting

In this example, we consider the case in which a clinical sample counted in an automatic gamma counter has two different radiopharmaceuticals present, and only one is intended to be counted. The most common clinical use for a gamma counter at present is in the counting of blood plasma samples as part of a radionuclide GFR test. Therefore, relevant clinical scenarios include those in which a patient has received two different radioactive administrations in relatively quick succession, such as [^{99m}Tc]-DMSA (dimercapto succinic acid) renal imaging followed by a [^{51}Cr]-EDTA (ethylenediaminetetraacetic acid) GFR test, or [^{177}Lu]-DOTATATE therapy followed by a [^{99m}Tc]-DTPA GFR test. In both of these cases, the activity administered during the GFR test is far less than that administered for the other diagnostic test or therapy. When GFR samples are counted using a gamma counter, the use of appropriate energy windows can assist in minimising the errors associated with counting multiple isotopes simultaneously.

The ARSAC diagnostic reference level (DRL) for a [^{51}Cr]-EDTA GFR is 3 MBq, compared to 80 MBq [^{99m}Tc]-DMSA for renal imaging, and ^{51}Cr has a 27.7-day half-life, which is significantly longer than that of ^{99m}Tc (0.25 days). If both tests are performed on the same day, the patient samples may be left to decay for an additional 48 h prior to counting, after which point the contribution from the ^{99m}Tc contaminant in the GFR samples will be negligible (<0.3% of its original contribution). In practical counting terms, this is also aided by the fact that the ^{99m}Tc energy peak at 140 keV is significantly lower than that of ^{51}Cr at 320 keV; therefore, scattered photons will not be observed in the higher-energy ^{51}Cr photopeak window.

In the other example, a [^{99m}Tc]-DTPA GFR (DRL = 10 MBq) occurs just after a [^{177}Lu]-DOTATATE therapy (typical administered activity = 7.4 GBq). The half-life of the ^{177}Lu is 6.65 days; therefore, if a significant amount of ^{177}Lu is present in the ^{99m}Tc GFR samples, decay storing the GFR samples will not work. Where clinically possible, the GFR test should therefore either be performed first, or alternatively be delayed until there is a sufficiently small amount of ^{177}Lu present in the blood compared to the ^{99m}Tc to be administered, such that only ^{99m}Tc photons are detectable in the subsequent blood sample. The amount of each radiopharmaceutical in the bloodstream changes as a function of time, given the biological uptake, excretion speed and pathway, and physical half-life of the isotope.

Let us examine the components of the spectra that could be acquired for a [^{99m}Tc]-DTPA sample when [^{177}Lu]-DOTATATE is also present. ^{177}Lu emits gamma rays at 55 keV (5%), 113 keV (6%), and 210 keV (11%) (Delacroix *et al* 2006).

The data in figure 10.7 was acquired on a HIDEX AMG automatic gamma counter. In this counter the preset energy window for ^{99m}Tc is 112–168 keV (i.e. a ±20% energy window around the photopeak), as demonstrated by the black vertical dashed lines. The solid black line shows the ^{99m}Tc spectrum between 0 and 400 keV

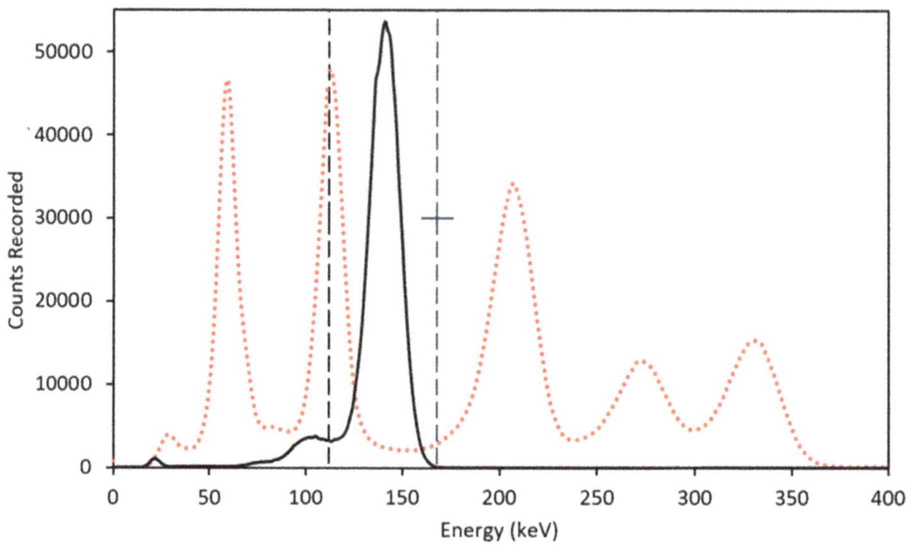

Figure 10.7. Gamma counter spectra for a ^{99m}Tc sample (solid black line) and a ^{177}Lu sample (dotted red line). The energy window for ^{99m}Tc in this counter is given by the two black dashed lines.

Table 10.4. Counts recorded for ^{99m}Tc and ^{177}Lu in the open energy window and a ^{99m}Tc energy window.

	Total counts in open energy window	Counts in ^{99m}Tc energy window
6 kBq ^{99m}Tc sample	1 189 268	1 089 268
15 kBq ^{177}Lu sample	3 827 682	552 586
1 kBq ^{99m}Tc	198 211	181 545
1 kBq ^{177}Lu	2 555 179	36 839

from a 3 mL sample containing ~6 kBq, and the red dotted line shows a spectrum from a 3 mL sample containing ~15 kBq ^{177}Lu. The relative counts acquired for the isotopes are shown in table 10.4.

Whilst the total counts per activity in the whole spectrum (15–2000 keV, more than is shown in figure 10.7) for ^{177}Lu are ~130% of those for ^{99m}Tc, the counts in the ^{99m}Tc energy window are ~5 times higher for ^{99m}Tc than for ^{177}Lu. In order to limit the extra counts from ^{177}Lu to ⩽1% of the counts in the ^{99m}Tc window, there would need to be ⩾20 times more ^{99m}Tc than ^{177}Lu in the sample, and the clinically administered activity ratio is 7400 MBq/10 MBq= 740 in favour of ^{177}Lu. Therefore, the GFR test should ideally be delayed after the [^{177}Lu]-DOTATATE administration for 14 [^{177}Lu]-DOTATATE effective half-lives in the blood. As a worst-case scenario, this would be a delay of 14 physical half-lives of ^{177}Lu, which is approximately three months. If this wait were unacceptable, one possible practical way to attempt to correct for the presence of ^{177}Lu in the [^{99m}Tc]-DPTA GFR sample would be as follows:

- Count the original samples and an original background sample;
- Background correct the original sample counts by subtracting the prompt background counts from the original sample counts;
- Re-count the samples and a delayed background approximately 72 h later, after which time the ^{99m}Tc component of the signal should be negligible (0.02% of the original ^{99m}Tc sample counts should remain);
- Background correct the delayed sample counts by subtracting the delayed background counts from the delayed sample counts;
- Decay correct the delayed background-corrected sample counts using the physical half-life of ^{177}Lu. Subtract this from the original background-corrected counts. The remaining counts should be a good approximation to the ^{99m}Tc counts in the original samples.

In order to ensure that there is <1% error due to purely statistical fluctuations, the counting times should be sufficient for at least 10 000 counts to be acquired in all samples for both the prompt and delayed samples. If this means that the delayed samples are counted for a different duration to that of the prompt ones, then this correction should also be included in the calculation.

An alternative numerical method for separating the contributions, in which the sensitivity to pure samples of each nuclide in both their respective energy windows is known for the counter, would be to use the technique described in section 9.7.2 'Dual radionuclide studies—general case'.

An additional consideration when one is attempting to isolate the counts from one radionuclide that is present in a mixture of radionuclides is the impact of the counts recorded by the counter outside the measurement energy window of the counter. This increases the dead time experienced by the counter. The impact of this may not be immediately obvious for counters which do not report the dead time within the measurement data visible to the user. It is also potentially more difficult to diagnose this situation when the second isotope only has scattered photons within the measurement window, and therefore there is a less significant impact on the counts recorded inside the measurement window itself. One example of this situation is an ^{18}F-based radiopharmaceutical contaminating a [^{99m}Tc]-DTPA GFR sample. Diagnosis of this problem could include routinely monitoring the dead time of the counter as patient samples are being counted and setting an appropriate local tolerance limit based on the counter and contamination isotopes. Alternatively, a wide or open energy window can be measured simultaneously with the clinical measurement energy window, to check on the overall measured counts per minute of the samples. A local limit may be set to indicate when the count rate in the open window is too high and dead time within the counter becomes significant; as a rough guide, this may be, for example, above 5 kcps. The full pulse height spectrum of any suspicious samples could be inspected for spurious peaks or to further investigate the origin of dead-time effects. In the case of ^{18}F contamination being detected, given its 1.83 h half-life, the ^{99m}Tc GFR samples could be counted >18 h later for a longer period to ensure that sufficient ^{99m}Tc counts are still measured. At this point, some of the ^{99m}Tc would still remain, but the ^{18}F should have (in practical terms) decayed (<0.1% of original administered activity remaining).

It is noted that for high-activity samples, the light pulses that reach the PMTs from the NaI(Tl) crystal arrive very rapidly, such that signals resulting from one gamma emission overlap with the next, causing a pulse pile-up (HIDEX 2017). This results in a shift of the spectrum towards higher energy, as the pulses are not distinguished as different and the signals are summed. Therefore, for high-activity samples, the pulse height spectrum is at a higher energy than for a low-activity sample. If this is the case, and the counter is not able to adequately correct for such an effect, where possible, the source should be allowed to decay prior to counting. Some modern counters can correct for this spectral shift, as described in section 4.4.3.

10.8 Worked example of sample volume effects on counting using a well counter

When deciding on the optimal sample volume to choose for a given purpose when using a gamma well counter, there are conflicting considerations that must be addressed. For a given activity concentration of an isotope, a larger sample will result in a linearly proportional greater number of emissions from the sample. In addition to this, for a given absolute pipetting error, the larger the sample, the smaller the fractional error in the volume of the sample. However, as discussed in section 4.6.13, well counter detectors suffer a loss of efficiency with increasing sample volume due to a reduction of geometric efficiency, as illustrated in figure 10.8.

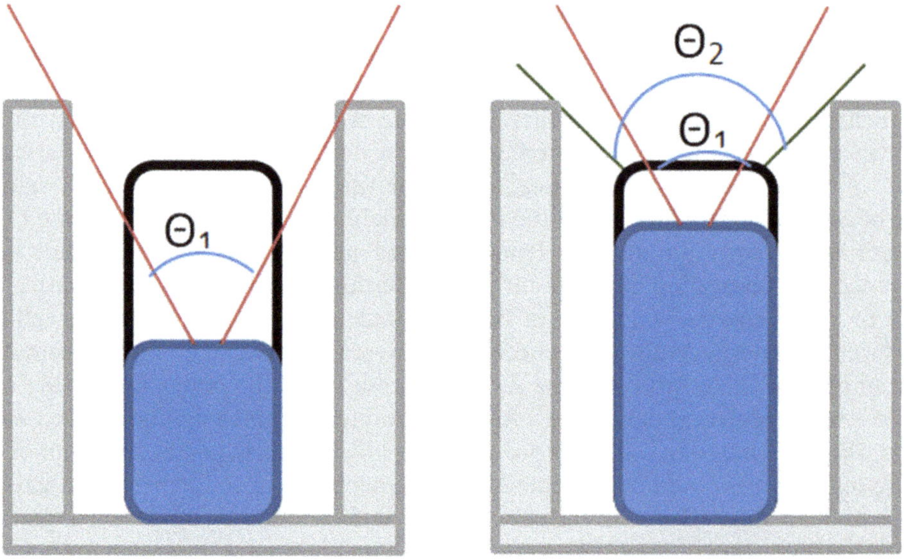

Figure 10.8. Loss of efficiency with increasing sample volume as a higher proportion of gamma rays escape the detector.

Also, in the case of higher-activity-concentration solutions, a larger sample may induce more significant dead-time effects in the counter.

Here, a worked example of sample volume impact on counter efficiency is provided for ^{99m}Tc, which illustrates the magnitude of these volume effects in a gamma well counter.

Multiple 0.5 mL identical samples were pipetted from the same standard of ^{99m}Tc with a sample activity <10 kBq to minimise dead-time effects. Each sample then had a different volume of water added to it, resulting in ten final samples containing the same activity but with volumes progressively increasing from 1 to 10 mL. Each sample was counted for 120 s to establish a low-noise reference count rate (Lodge *et al* 2015). Figure 10.9 illustrates the measured sample counts plotted against sample volume for the ten samples. The relative efficiency of ^{99m}Tc reduces as a function of sample volume with a faster reduction rate for higher sample volumes, representing higher geometric count losses as the sample volume reaches the top of the well counter.

It is therefore preferential overall to optimise the sample volume for a particular counting scenario by considering:

- the sample volume available;
- the sample volume required to provide good count statistics;
- the total activity contained within the sample to ensure that dead-time effects are not significant; and
- the impact of differences (or errors) in the pipetted sample volume in terms of changes in geometric counting efficiency of the well counter.

Figure 10.8 demonstrates the impact of sample volume on geometric efficiency for counting. As the sample size increases, a higher proportion of the gamma rays

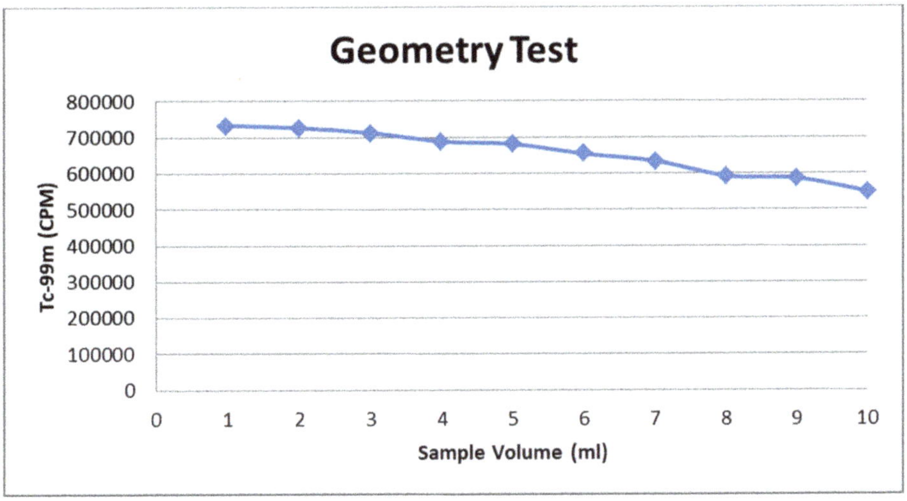

Figure 10.9. Plot showing the sensitivity change of the counter with volume.

emitted escape from the well without interacting with the detector, as the relative solid angle of the detector from the sample reduces (as is shown by $\theta_1 < \theta_2$).

Figure 10.9 demonstrates a practical example of how this translates into a relative reduction in the counts measured over a set time, given constant activity samples of varying volumes. Based on figures 10.8 and 10.9, it is recommended to avoid using particularly small sample volumes, in order to ensure that that the overall count measured is high whilst not causing significant dead time, albeit with reduced geometric efficiency. For example, a 3 mL plasma sample from a [^{99m}Tc]-DTPA GFR would give approximately 5.86 times more counts than a 0.5 mL plasma sample when both the activity contained and volume effects are considered. A 3 mL plasma volume is normally achievable from commonly used clinical blood tubes without the need to top up samples with water. Counts from a patient sample such as this would not be expected to cause problematic dead-time effects in a clinical gamma counter. The additional benefit of the larger sample lies in its smaller fractional error from pipetting inaccuracies. Here, a 0.05 mL pipetting error results in a 10% error in a 0.5 mL sample, compared to only a 1.7% error in a 3 mL sample.

10.9 Worked example of blood sample counting for therapy dosimetry

Blood dosimetry can be used in clinical practice for radionuclide therapy planning, such as for ^{131}I therapy for differentiated thyroid cancer and in the research environment for evaluating clearance patterns of novel radiopharmaceuticals (Lassmann *et al* 2008). For radiopharmaceuticals that bind to blood products and the red marrow, blood sampling is essential for blood dosimetry.

This section presents an example of blood dosimetry performed using ^{111}In-antibody (anti-cd66) as part of planning for radioimmunotherapy with ^{90}Y-antibody. This radiopharmaceutical binds to blood cells and red marrow and is used for bone marrow ablation prior to stem cell engraftment. Blood sampling is performed to evaluate the blood clearance rate on an individual patient basis and to improve red marrow dose estimation (Hindorf *et al* 2010).

Following the administration of 185 MBq of ^{111}In-antibody, 5 mL whole-blood samples in EDTA tubes were taken at 0, 1, 2, 4, 24, 72, and 96 h and stored at 4 °C. At the end of the sampling period, the blood samples were gently mixed and duplicate 1 mL samples from each timepoint were pipetted into counting tubes. Additionally, standard samples were prepared by diluting 6 MBq ^{111}In in 1000 mL distilled water, mixing thoroughly, and pipetting duplicate 1 mL samples.

The samples and standards were counted using a dual detector well counter system. A single energy window was selected from 150–280 keV to cover both gamma emissions of ^{111}In (171 and 245 keV). Because these two gammas are emitted almost simultaneously, a summation peak at about 416 keV was also observed. This summation peak would potentially be useful if the counter is located in an area where the background can vary during the counting period due to nearby transit of lower-energy high-activity radioactive sources (e.g., ^{99m}Tc). Alternatively, a wide energy window from 100–500 keV can be used to additionally include the summation peak of ^{111}In, providing improved sensitivity in measurement (Pai-Scherf *et al* 2000).

The counting time was chosen to be 100s, which ensured minimum total counts >10 000 in the lowest activity (96 h) sample, yielding a 1% error assuming Poisson statistics.

Blank counting tubes for background correction were counted immediately before and after counting the samples.

The resulting counts were background corrected and normalised against the counts of the ^{111}In standard to calculate the activity contained in each sample. The sample activities were plotted against the sample time to create a time–activity curve for antibody clearance from blood, as shown in the log–linear diagram in figure 10.10. A three-phase exponential curve was fitted, which outlined a rapid blood clearance pattern in the first few hours post administration, followed by slower clearance with an effective half-life of 31 h from the first day post administration onwards. This blood clearance curve was then used to evaluate the dose to the bone marrow and determine the required activity of ^{90}Y-antibody to achieve bone marrow ablation, while staying within dose limits, to enable successful stem cell engraftment post ablation.

The blood clearance curve can be used for bone marrow dosimetry. For radiopharmaceuticals that have no specific uptake in bone marrow cells, the activity in the bone marrow can be directly estimated from the blood activity concentration and the patient's heamatocrit without the need for patient imaging. However, in cases in which there is specific radiopharmaceutical uptake in bone marrow cells,

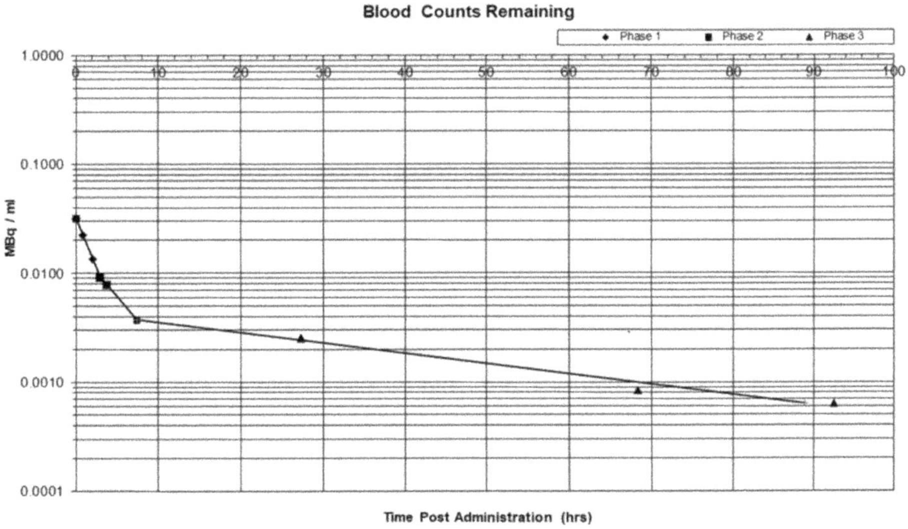

Figure 10.10. ^{111}In-antibody time–activity curve indicating rapid clearance from blood.

quantitative imaging is required for bone marrow dosimetry as outlined in the European Association of Nuclear Medicine (EANM) Guidelines (Hindorf *et al* 2010).

10.10 Worked example of the use of Shewhart and CUSUM control charts

These example data were obtained from a sodium iodide-based gamma counter measuring a solid ^{137}Cs source. The total counts (peak area) are recorded in a fixed gamma energy window around the main photopeak for ^{137}Cs (662 keV) with a measurement time of 2000 s. The observed counts are corrected for dead time, decay (to a common reference time), and background and are divided by the measurement time to give counts per second.

The first 16 measurements shown in table 10.5 are the 'control' data. The mean and standard deviation of the data were determined and used to calculate the upper and lower warning (3σ) and control (2σ) limits shown below in figure 10.11. The difference between each measurement and the mean was calculated, and the CUSUM was determined by sequentially summing these differences, as plotted in figure 10.12.

Measurements 17–19 are independent of the control data and are plotted alongside the control data without modifying the mean, the standard deviation, or the control limits.

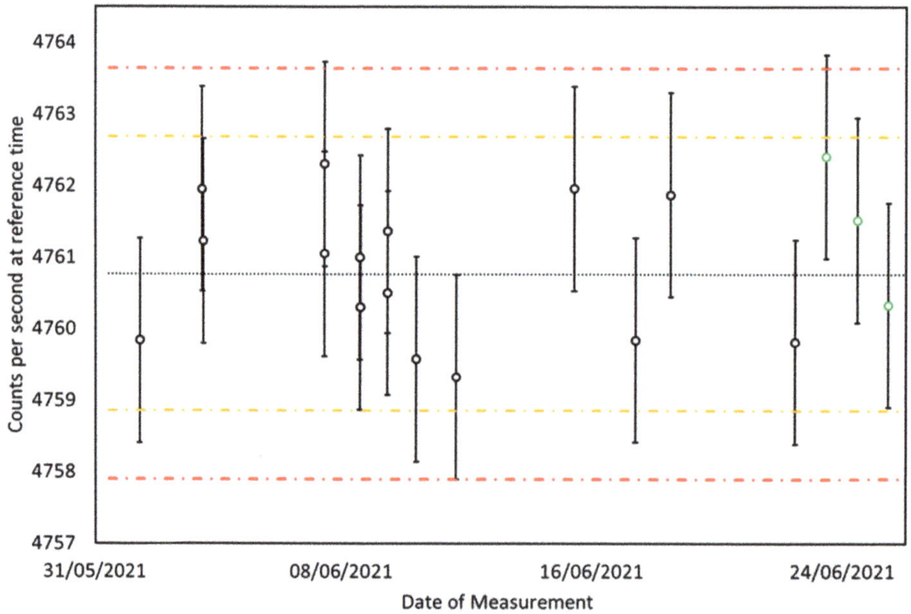

Figure 10.11. Shewhart chart using example data. Red lines indicate control limits, yellow lines indicate warning limits, and green points are the measurement data plotted after the calculation of the control limits.

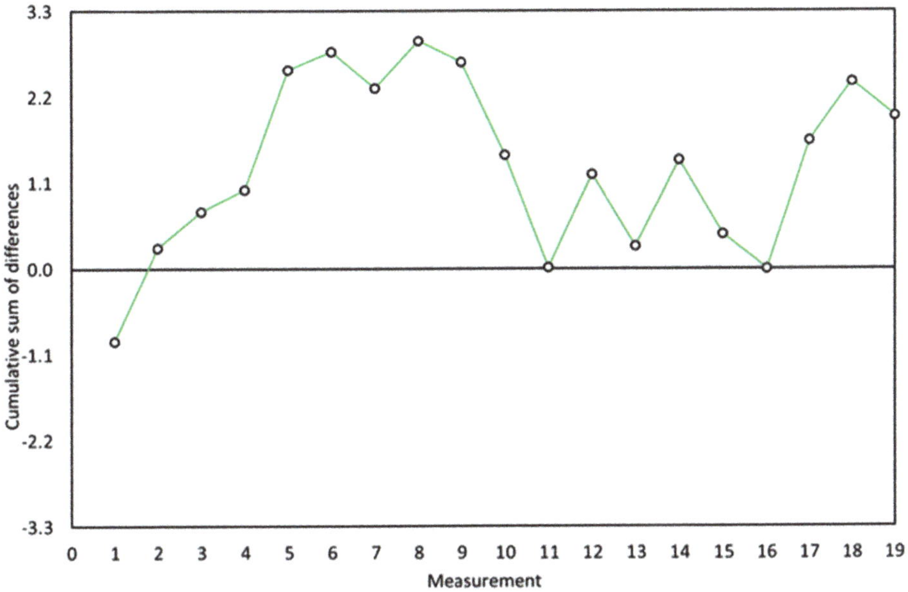

Figure 10.12. CUSUM chart using the same example data as those used for the Shewhart chart.

Table 10.5. Control and measurement data used for quality control of a gamma counter.

Measurement number	Measurement date	Counts per second (at reference time)	Difference	CUSUM
1	01/06/2021 10:43	4759.8	−0.9	−0.9
2	03/06/2021 11:35	4762.0	1.2	0.3
3	03/06/2021 12:29	4761.2	0.5	0.7
4	07/06/2021 11:12	4761.0	0.3	1.0
5	07/06/2021 11:24	4762.3	1.5	2.5
6	08/06/2021 14:17	4761.0	0.2	2.8
7	08/06/2021 14:30	4760.3	−0.5	2.3
8	09/06/2021 11:07	4761.4	0.6	2.9
9	09/06/2021 11:22	4760.5	−0.3	2.6
10	10/06/2021 09:18	4759.6	−1.2	1.5
11	11/06/2021 16:14	4759.3	−1.4	0.0
12	15/06/2021 09:56	4762.0	1.2	1.2
13	17/06/2021 09:23	4759.8	−0.9	0.3
14	18/06/2021 12:30	4761.9	1.1	1.4
15	22/06/2021 11:50	4759.8	−1.0	0.4
16	22/06/2021 12:56	4760.3	−0.4	0.0

Mean	4760.8
Standard deviation	1.0
Upper warning limit	4762.7
Upper control limit	4763.6
Lower warning limit	4758.9
Lower control limit	4757.9

Measurement number	Measurement date	Counts per second (at reference time)	Difference	CUSUM
17	23/06/2021 11:11	4762.4	1.6	1.6
18	24/06/2021 10:50	4761.5	0.8	2.4
19	25/06/2021 10:36	4760.3	−0.4	2.0

References

Amor-Coarasa A, Schoendorf M, Meckel M, Vallabhajosula S and Babich J W 2016 Comprehensive quality control of the ITG 68Ge/68Ga generator and synthesis of 68Ga-DOTATOC and 68Ga-PSMA-HBED-CC for clinical imaging *J. Nucl. Med.* **57** 1402–405

Burniston M 2018 *Clinical Guideline for the Measurement of Glomerular Filtration Rate (GFR) Using Plasma Sampling* (London: British Nuclear Medicine Society)

Cunningham V J, Gunn R N and Matthews J C 2004 Quantification in positron emission tomography for research in pharmacology and drug development *Nucl. Med. Commun.* **25** 643–46

Delacroix D, Guerre J P and Leblanc P 2006 Guide Pratique Radionuclides & Radioprotection 2nd edn (Société Francaise de Radioprotection)

Green M A, Mathias C J and Fletcher J W 2016 Experience in production of 68Ga-DOTA-NOC for clinical use under an expanded access IND *Appl. Radiat. Isot.* **116** 63–8

HIDEX Automatic Gamma Counter User Guide, Software Version 1.2.16.0 2017

Hindorf C, Glatting G, Chiesa C, Lindén O and Flux G 2010 EANM Dosimetry Committee guidelines for bone marrow and whole-body dosimetry *Eur. J. Nucl. Med. Mol. Imaging* **37** 1238–250

Lassmann M, Hänscheid H, Chiesa C, Hindorf C, Flux G and Luster M 2008 EANM Dosimetry Committee series on standard operational procedures for pre-therapeutic dosimetry I: blood and bone marrow dosimetry in differentiated thyroid cancer therapy *Eur. J. Nucl. Med. Mol. Imaging* **35** 1405

Lodge M A, Holt D P, Kinahan P E, Wong D F and Wahl R L 2015 Performance assessment of a NaI (Tl) gamma counter for PET applications with methods for improved quantitative accuracy and greater standardization *EJNMMI Phys* **2** 11

Morris E D *et al* 2004 Kinetic modeling in positron emission tomography *Emission Tomography* (Amsterdam: Elsevier) 499–540

Oikonen V 2011 Introduction to Modelling, Turku PET Symposium, http://www.turkupetcentre.net/petanalysis/modelling_intro.html, Last Updated 8/12/2018, Last Visited 27/5/2022

Pai-Scherf L H *et al* 2000 Imaging and phase I study of 111In-and 90Y-labeled anti-LewisY monoclonal antibody B3 *Clin. Cancer Res.* **6** 1720–30

Turku PET Centre *Reliable Blood Data for Full PET Quantification, PMOD Application Note* PMOD Technologies LLC 2019 http://www.turkupetcentre.net/petanalysis/modelling_intro.html)

Vis R, Lavalaye J and van de Garde E M 2015 GMP-compliant 68 Ga radiolabelling in a conventional small-scale radiopharmacy: a feasible approach for routine clinical use *EJNMMI Res* **5** 27

Appendix A

Troubleshooting gamma counters

Problem encountered	Potential reason(s)	Troubleshooting steps
High background counts	• Contaminated well. • Contaminated workbench/conveyor. • Source of external radiation. • Faulty detector.	• Check for contamination and decontaminate well or workbench/conveyor, as necessary. • Check for potential sources of external radiation such as waste, other sample tubes, sealed sources, or radioactive patients located nearby. • Check order of samples. • Repeat background tests with open window after performing the above steps. • Check spectra for unexpected peaks.
Low efficiency	• Incorrect source activity entered during calibration • Incorrect isotope used • Faulty detector	• Check the activity written on the tube • Replace detector
Zero counts	• Incorrect count time • High background value • Incorrect isotope selected	• Check count time and isotope on protocol settings • Disable background subtraction

doi:10.1088/978-0-7503-3895-0ch11

Appendix B

Troubleshooting gamma probes

Below is a basic troubleshooting guide for problems that may be found during testing, such as the daily QC of intraoperative gamma probes. Its aim is to provide a simple guide to possible reasons why the probe is not performing as expected. It is not an exhaustive list, and in the event that the situation encountered is not solved here, the reader is recommended to seek further advice from the relevant Medical Physics Expert and/or the probe manufacturer.

Problem encountered	Possible causes and/or solutions
Detected counts far higher than expected	• Probe on wrong energy window (e.g. may be wider than normally used). Change to correct window and repeat test. • Probe has wrong/no collimator present during measurement. Repeat measurement with correct collimator. • Distance from probe to source is too small. Repeat at correct testing distance. • Counts measured in area of high background. Check background and test in area with lower background. • Probe contaminated. Decontaminate and repeat measurement. • Incorrect test source is being used (higher activity than expected). Repeat test with correct source. • Counting time is greater than expected. Adjust to required value and repeat test. • If multiple probe system, wrong probe selected on base unit. Repeat test with correct probe selected.

(*Continued*)

doi:10.1088/978-0-7503-3895-0ch12

(*Continued*)

Problem encountered	Possible causes and/or solutions
Detected counts/count rates slightly higher or lower than expected	• Probe on wrong energy window. Change to correct window and repeat test. • Probe has wrong collimator present during measurement. Repeat measurement with correct collimator. • Distance from probe to source incorrect. Repeat at correct testing distance. • Counts measured in area of some background. Check background and test in area with lower background. • Counts measured close to metal surface or alternatively high-scatter surface, causing backscatter of photons measured by probe. Repeat measurement away from scattering surface. • Check the orientation of probe in which the counts were acquired. Some probes may measure slightly different counts when they are held in different orientations. • If the test is being performed with the jig held sideways, with the probe resting along the table, the probe tip might not be in contact with the source, and therefore the distance to the source will be slightly bigger and then QC counts will be slightly low. Hold jig with probe in vertical orientation and repeat test. • Check whether the source is in the correct orientation in the jig. Sealed radioactive disc sources which are usually used for daily quality control testing have their activity closer to one flat side than the other, therefore the orientation in the test jig impacts on the probe-to-source distance during testing. Flip the source over in the jig and repeat the test. • In wired systems, coiling of the measurement cables can produce spurious electrical effects. • If the original baseline measurements were acquired when probe was suffering non-negligible dead time, then the apparent sensitivity will gradually increase. This may happen when the original count rates were >1000cps, but the count rate for which dead time is significant is probe dependent, and ideally would be determined during acceptance testing. Depending on the frequency at which testing takes place, i.e. if the probe is not tested for months or more, it may appear to cause a step change in sensitivity. In this eventuality, and assuming no other problems with the probe are suspected, QC limits should be regenerated regularly as the source decays to account for the reduction in dead time.

	• If multiple probe system, wrong probe selected on base unit. Repeat test with correct probe selected.
If counts/count rates are significantly lower than expected	• For systems that require internal calibration daily, the calibration has not been done or has failed. Repeat calibration and test again. • Perform a visual check—is probe or its cabling damaged/visibly cracked? Does the reading noticeably fluctuate as the probe/cable are moved? If so, contact the manufacturer, as repair may be required. • Probe on wrong energy window. Change to correct window and repeat test. • Probe has wrong collimator present during measurement. Repeat measurement with correct collimator. • Distance from probe to source too large. Repeat at correct testing distance. • Incorrect test source is being used (lower activity than expected). Repeat test with correct source. • Counting time is smaller than expected. Adjust to required value and repeat test.
If the readings for the source or background have high variability	• For wired systems, the cable or connectors could be damaged. This can be tested by gently manually manipulating the cable in the absence of sources, near to where it connects to the probe, in the middle, and near to the base unit, and see whether any spurious counts appear. Any spurious counts may indicate that the cable needs replacement and could account for low counts. • For Bluetooth systems, there may be electrical interference with other equipment/mobile phones. Retest away from other equipment and phones. • For Bluetooth systems, capacitive effects in the probe may cause spurious signals. Try moving the probe around or touching it in different places to diagnose this. If this is suspected, probe is likely to require a manufacturer repair.
Probe fails to measure any counts	• If multiple probe system, wrong probe selected on base unit. Repeat test with correct probe selected. • Probe is not properly assembled and powered. Check probe setup and repeat test. • Incorrect jig used. Repeat test with correct setup.

(*Continued*)

(*Continued*)

Problem encountered	Possible causes and/or solutions
	• Test source not present in jig. Repeat test with correct setup. • Incorrect energy window selected. Adjust to correct window and repeat test. • Poor connection in the probe or cable may be preventing measurement. If available, a different cable/probe could be tested with the base unit to diagnose this. This may require repair by manufacturer, therefore contact them for more advice. • Probe on wrong energy window. Change to correct window and repeat test.

www.ingramcontent.com/pod-product-compliance
Ingram Content Group UK Ltd.
Pitfield, Milton Keynes, MK11 3LW, UK
UKHW051850100926
8556IPUK00005B/551

9 780750 338936